Pocket Field Guide for Disaster Health Professionals

David A. Bradt
Christina M. Drummond

Pocket Field Guide for Disaster Health Professionals

Missioncraft in Disaster Relief® Series

Springer

DMCIS
Missioncraft in Disaster Relief

David A. Bradt
Baltimore, MD
USA

Christina M. Drummond
Melbourne, VIC
Australia

ISBN 978-3-030-04800-6 ISBN 978-3-030-04801-3 (eBook)
https://doi.org/10.1007/978-3-030-04801-3

This Springer imprint is published by the registered company Springer Nature Switzerland AG
The registered company address is: Gewerbestrasse 11, 6330 Cham, Switzerland

This Field Guide is dedicated to the humanitarian aid workers, including local staff, who have lost their lives serving others and to those who labor in the field with little safety, security, comfort, or thanks.

Acknowledgments

We wish to acknowledge the mentors, teachers, and colleagues who have taught us our craft. These black belt operators have collectively saved the lives of countless thousands of people and helped save ours as well. We are eternally in their debt.

Field

Tom Durant*—Cambodia, Zaire, Macedonia
Bob Brenner—Pakistan, Laos, Peru
Peter Galpin—places dark and scary
Judy Lee—USA
Luis Jorge Perez—Indonesia, India
Pino Annunziata—Indonesia, Tunisia
Johanna Larusdottir—India, Sri Lanka
Eigil Sorensen—Indonesia, India
Kate Farnsworth—Sudan
Andre Kisselev—Zaire
Keith Bentley—Indonesia
Tom Dolan—Indonesia
Nawal Osman—Sudan
Haider Abu Ahmed—Sudan
AK Siddique—Bangladesh
Marguerite Ryle*—USA
Jim Ellis*—Cambodia

Headquarters of governmental, non-governmental, Red Cross, and UN organizations

(Individuals are identified with their institutional affiliation during formative periods of interaction with the authors. Cited affiliations are not necessarily current.)

Skip Burkle—Harvard Humanitarian Initiative
Tim Baker*—Johns Hopkins University School of Public Health
Sue Baker—Johns Hopkins University School of Public Health
Allen Yung*—Fairfield Infectious Diseases Hospital
Pierre Perrin—International Committee of the Red Cross

Rudi Coninx—International Committee of the Red Cross
Claude de Ville de Goyet—Pan-American Health Organization
Helene Monteil—American Red Cross International Services
Jorge Castilla—World Health Organization
Fred Cuny*—Intertech
Peter Wallis—USAID Office of US Foreign Disaster Assistance
Mike VanRooyen—Johns Hopkins University School of Medicine

* In memoriam

We are grateful to the following foundations and societies for their assistance during critical phases of this work:

The Rockefeller Foundation
John Simon Guggenheim Memorial Foundation
Australasian Society for Infectious Diseases

We thank Peter Galpin, Amanda Norton, and Jonathan Robinson of the Disaster Medical Coordination International Society for their guidance, encouragement, and enduring support.

Contents

Introduction

Pocket Field Guide for Disaster Health Professionals: Missioncraft in Disaster Relief is written for full-time, field-based, hands-on health professionals serving in disaster relief operations. Disaster health professionals are burdened with data overload, information poverty, and the relentless pace of just-in-time decision-making. They must possess the technical competence to render an informed opinion, the administrative authority to mobilize resources, and the organizational responsibility for outcomes. They need a rich, portable fund of knowledge and state-of-the-art tools. This *Field Guide* focuses on their needs. It provides simple and versatile instruments for multitasking health professionals working under tight deadlines in urgent settings. The goal is to help standardize and improve professional practice—especially for disaster health coordinators. The *Field Guide* is not intended for medical tourists.

Organization of the Field Guide

The *Field Guide* is designed to be carried and used in the disaster setting. It is **organized to assist with key field activities—field briefing, field assessment, field recommendations, field reporting, field project and staff management, medical coordination, and reentry.** Each activity domain is addressed in a dedicated section of the *Field Guide*. Sections are sequenced as above to align with the chronological order of generic steps in disaster relief operations. Hence, information derived from one section may inform actions arising from the next section. For example, assessment informs recommendations which inform initial reporting and subsequent project design. Individual sections may also be used as needed to address issues spontaneously arising in the field.

Individual sections contain concise, comprehensive data gathering templates and associated reference data. The templates are self-contained, portable, and formatted for immediate use. They are data-dense and written in outline format—with indicator, space for field data, and reference benchmark. Overall, the documents function as minimum essential datasets (MEDS). These MEDS enable the user to arrive at an early, accurate picture of the health situation in the field. MEDS are sufficiently detailed to be authoritative, sufficiently brief to be manageable, and sufficiently useful to inform most common decisions made about health programs in the field.

Technical Annexes are repositories of core technical information located in Section 7. Acronyms are extensively listed in the last Annex.

Application

Do no harm. Beware of malpractice in disaster relief operations:

- Programmatic decisions without multiparty needs assessment
- Programmatic interventions without beneficiary input
- Non-reporting/non-sharing of local epidemiological data
- Nonparticipation in health sector/cluster coordination processes
- Health services without environmental health
- Clinical care without proper medical waste disposal
- Noncompliance with standardized case management
- Early primary closure for contaminated traumatic wounds
- Antidepressants for PTSD diagnosed in the field
- Introduction of unsustainable technology
- Establishment of refugee camps
- Population abandonment (under cover of "program transfer" to local health authorities) once international media leave and funding ends
- Glowing reports of program success which rely on process indicators without impact/outcome indicators

Data are not created equal. Many indicators exist for any given subject, and they have different sources, acquisition methods, availabilities, utilities, costs, and technical limitations. This *Field Guide* does not detail these issues but rather makes an explicit judgment about indicator usefulness through de facto inclusion in datasets. Moreover, providers are not trained equal. We do not explain indicators in this *Field Guide*. We simply use them to help characterize the professional practice of disaster relief specialists.

It is understood that not all data points, even in a MEDS framework, are needed to inform field decisions. Small amounts of reliable, relevant data will usually suffice. Medical coordinators may choose to customize the templates with indicators and benchmarks most relevant to their agency. Some programmatic decisions, in particular specialty areas (e.g., immunization programs, feeding programs), may require additional data gathered thru dedicated surveys or disease surveillance beyond the scope of this *Field Guide*.

Unless stated otherwise, masculine nouns and pronouns in the *Field Guide* refer to both genders.

Feedback

Disaster health professionals work in the "field." The field is not the capital city or country office. It is often not even the field office. The field is where the beneficiaries are found. Ground truth comes from the deep field. The way to do important work is to work on important things. Disaster health professionals undertake important things in urgent settings. They will be the ultimate judges of the usefulness of the *Field Guide*. To that end, feedback from experienced users is welcomed at info@dmcis.org.

1 Field Briefing

Contents

Overview

This section provides guidance on field briefing. Briefing is one of the weakest parts of professional practice in the disaster health sector. Headquarters and regional offices often lack detailed knowledge about the field and commonly refer incoming health personnel with specific questions to the field. Once in the field, health personnel may find their predecessors have already left. When overlap does occur, briefings in the acute disaster setting may be rushed and ad hoc. Standardized handover protocols are rarely used. Just as shift change can harm patients in emergency departments and hospital wards, so can shift change harm beneficiaries in disaster health programs. Ultimately, a bad handover is the bane of the receiver. Once the incumbent leaves the field, the successor owns the problem whether he knows about it or not. Whether you are first in the field, or next to last, briefing is a leadership opportunity to bring order to chaos.

This section focuses on 2 major briefing issues—safety/security and health status.

- Safety/security—encompasses 3 key domains
  - Comprehensive safety and security plan
  - Subordinate component plans—communications, medevac, contingency, and evacuation

D. A. Bradt, C. M. Drummond, *Pocket Field Guide for Disaster Health Professionals*,
https://doi.org/10.1007/978-3-030-04801-3_1

- SOPS—security updates, activities of daily living, communications, travel, and routine notifications

Noncompliance with security procedures is cause for summary dismissal from the field.

- Health status—encompasses 8 key domains
  - Scope of work and terms of reference
  - Agency background and work environment
  - Host country government and health system
  - Beneficiaries
  - Incident management
  - Cluster process
  - Project management
  - Normative technical practices

Document 1.1
SECURITY CHECKLIST

Safety & Security Officer

Name

Contact details

Emergency services phone #s

Safety and Security Plan (SSP)

Plan	Received (Y/N)	Obtain From
SSP comprehensive		
Comms Plan		
Medevac Plan		
Contingency Plans		
Evacuation Plan		
SOPs	**Received (Y/N)**	**Obtain From**
Security update		
Activities of Daily Living		
Comms (primary, alternate, contingency, & emergency)		
Travel (primary, alternate, contingency, & emergency)		
Routine check-in/notifications		

Current Situation ETHANE	**Tactical Situation METT-T**	**Operations Orders SMEAC**
Exact location (of incident)	**M**ission	**S**ituation
Type of incident (hazard)	**E**nemy	**M**ission
Hazards present	**T**errain	**E**xecution
Access for emergency vehicles	**T**roops	**A**dmin & logistics
Number & severity of casualties	**T**ime available	**C**ommand & signals
Emergency services present & needed		

Document 1.1
ORIENTATION TO THE OFFICE

Find building entry/exit points.

Find landlines and sat phones.

Find smoke detectors, fire alarms, and fire extinguishers.

Find smoke hoods, hard hats, and flashlights.

Find first aid kit.

Find protected room for shelter-in-place. Otherwise, find toilet block (often structurally sounder than main building with ventilation and water source).

Find building escape route and outside rally point.

Find escape routes from the neighborhood.

Get GPS coordinates for office and home. Know 3 routes between them.

Know how to call the security officer, neighborhood warder, team leader, and phone tree contacts.

Document 1.2
MEDICAL HANDOVER CHECKLIST

A. Scope of Work/Terms of Reference

1. Responsibilities
   a. key deliverables
2. Authorities (#1 and #2 must be compatible)
   a. staff
   b. material (comms, vehicles)
   c. financial (accounts, cash)
3. Reporting requirements—to whom, how often, what level of detail

B. Agency Background and Work Environment

1. Mission statement and host country permission to operate
2. Organogram
3. Contact lists
4. Administrative rules
   a. staff support (secretarial, logistics)
   b. key policies (eg security, resource management, media)
   c. travel authorization & security clearance
   d. length of assignment
   e. work week, pay schedule
   f. benefits—insurance, liability limits
5. Security plan, security briefing
   a. security officer address, contact details
   b. warden address, contact details
6. Communications plan, comms briefing
   a. radio room location, contact details
7. Medical evacuation plan, health briefing
   a. medical facility location, contact details
8. Work processes and products
   a. correspondence
      1. e-mail address
      2. list serves
   b. reporting
      1. sitreps (monthly)
      2. cluster bulletins (monthly)
      3. EWARN reports (weekly)
      4. epidemic-specific reports (ad hoc)
      5. maps
   c. archives
      1. shared drives
      2. google docs (invitation)
9. Office address, contact details
10. Home address, contact details

C. Host Country Government and Health System

1. Country profile (eg DCI factbook)
2. Health system profile
3. Public health profile (eg WHO Communicable Disease Profile)
4. Emergency management system profile
5. MOH organogram
6. Current government appeals
7. Status of relationships

D. Beneficiaries

1. Local map (1:100,000)
2. Local map with camp locations
3. Table of # refugees and # HoH by (sub)districts
4. Table of # refugee sites by (sub)districts and site population size bracket (< 5,000, 5,000-10,000, 10,000–15,000 etc)
5. Table of # refugee sites and # refugees by health center catchments
6. Quantitation of vulnerable groups—U5, orphaned, pregnant, etc
7. Status of relationships

E. Incident Management

1. Organogram
2. Job action sheets, position task books
3. Local (country) office repurposing plan
4. Staff succession plan and absences from key positions
5. Incident action plan
6. Delegated authorities (finance)
7. Upcoming deliverables in humanitarian program cycle and emergency response framework

F. Cluster Process

1. Partners and key contacts
2. 4 Ws (who-what-where-when or area-activity matrix)
3. HeRAMS
4. Gap analysis—qualitative assessment of unmet need
5. Integrated subsector planning (pairing of iNGOs with local NGOs and health structures)
6. Strategic response plan
7. Multi-party (added value) actions in hazard mitigation, vulnerability reduction
8. Status of relationships

G. Project Management

1. Key strategy documents
2. Project plans of action
3. Periodic progress reports—copies (hard and soft) of last 3 monthly medical reports with instructions on locating original source documents from which the reports were compiled

4. Other work product
   a. assessments
   b. appeals
   c. evaluations
   d. prevention-preparedness-mitigation-response plans
5. Human resources documents
   a. project organogram
   b. weekly schedule of internal and external meetings to attend
   c. future staff needs
6. Material resources documents
   a. logistics assets and allocation
   b. current shortages in critical goods
   c. inventory of warehoused commodities
7. Financial resources documents
   a. donor alert
   b. flash appeal
   c. regional office funds available
   d. headquarters funds available
8. Key documentation—existing contracts, MOUs, correspondence
9. List of issues which will need attention or explode within the first week on the job—and analysis of those issues
10. List of correspondence which will need reply within the first week on the job
11. Health sector status summary
12. Assessment of current problems in non-clinical sectors which impact medical care
    a. security
    b. logistics
    c. environmental health—water, food, sanitation, shelter, vector control
    d. preventive medicine—labs to confirm index cases of epidemics, vaccine stocks

H. Normative Technical Practices

1. Standardized case management
   a. clinical case definitions
   b. treatment protocols authorized by MOH in host country
   c. other clinical protocols (standard precautions, injection safety, medical waste mgmt)
   d. essential drugs and rational drug use
   e. secondary prevention
   f. referral guidelines
2. Epidemiological surveillance
   a. clinical case definitions
   b. site recording sheets
   c. weekly surveillance report forms

   d. analysis and reporting process—description and diagram
   e. responsible official
   f. recent field studies
3. Epidemic preparedness
   a. list of disease outbreaks and epidemic threats
   b. plan of action
   c. clinical case definitions (especially if differ from surveillance definition)
   d. case management guidelines for communicable diseases with epidemic potential
   e. outbreak management protocol
   f. secondary prevention
   g. resource prepositioning and stockpiles
   h. information management
   i. contingency planning
4. Other

I. Meetings Schedule

1. Local agency
2. Health cluster
3. Inter-cluster working group
4. Regional office and headquarters teleconferences

J. Contact List (office address, phone, and contact list)

1. Index organization
2. Government officials
3. UN, IOs
4. NGOs
5. Focal points for document distribution

Document 1.3
HEALTH SYSTEM PROFILE

I. CONTEXT

A. Legal Framework

B. Rights Framework (to health care)

C. Social Participation and Control

II. POLITICAL JURISDICTIONS

III. INDICATORS

A. Access to Essential Services (see UNICEF [1], WHO [2])

1. Public utilities (infrastructure)
   a. % population with access to improved water
   b. % population with access to improved sanitation
   c. % population with electricity
   d. % population with telephones/television
2. Health services
   a. skilled health care workers (doctor + nurse + midwife etc)/10,000 p (23)
   b. physicians/10,000 p
   c. nurses/10,000 p
   d. community health workers/10,000 p (10)
   e. % population with provider coverage (100%)
   f. consultations/p/yr (1)
   g. % pregnancies receiving antenatal care (100%)
   h. % deliveries attended by trained staff (90%)
   i. % immunization rates—measles vac in 1 y/o (90%)
   j. hospital beds/10,000 p (10)
   k. health facilities with BEOC, CEOC/500,000 p (4, 1)
   l. admissions/10,000 p
3. Underserved areas (by location and type of service)

B. Health Status (see UNICEF [1], WHO [2])

1. Mortality and other rates
   a. CBR (10–50)
   b. CMR (5–25)
   c. AGR (%)
   d. IMR (3–200)
   e. U5MR (3–300)
   f. MMR (5–2,100)

g. E_0 at birth M/F/T (40–85)
h. TFR (2–8)

2. Nutritional status
   a. caloric intake/p/d (2,100 kcal)
   b. % infants with low birth weight (LBW) (7% with < 2.5 kg)
   c. % U5 with growth faltering (30%)
   d. % U5 with global acute malnutrition (GAM) (10%)
   e. % with micronutrient deficiencies (vitamins A-D; Fe, I)
   f. % of food supply from international food assistance (WFP, NGOs)
3. Endemic diseases
   a. HIV prevalence
   b. TB prevalence
   c. malaria incidence
   d. other major diseases
4. Health beliefs and traditions
5. Sources of care
6. Referral system

IV. SYSTEM DESCRIPTION

A. Public Health Services

1. Disease prevention
   a. primary prevention
      (1) vaccine coverage rates for major antigens (EPI coverage rate > 90%)
         (a) measles
         (b) DPT
      (2) vaccine stocks quantity available location
         (a) measles
         (b) DPT
         (c) polio
         (d) hepatitis B
         (e) other
      (3) cold chain adequacy
      (4) staff adequacy
      (5) transport adequacy
      (6) most recent campaign in area
         (a) location
         (b) dates
         (c) organizer
         (d) coverage
      (7) other VPIs of epidemic potential
   b. communicable disease control programs Y/N issues
      (1) diarrhea
      (2) ARI
      (3) malaria

(4) HIV
(5) TB
(6) other

2. Epidemiological surveillance system (CDC [3])
   a. system objectives
      (1) case detection (CDs, NCDs eg malnutrition)
      (2) outbreak detection
      (3) epidemic forecasting
      (4) trend monitoring
      (5) priority setting
      (6) workload estimation
      (7) resource targeting & health program activity
      (8) intervention evaluation
   b. health events/indicator conditions and case definitions
   c. system components and flow chart of operations
      (1) what is the population under surveillance?
      (2) what is the time period of data collection?
      (3) what data are collected (standardized forms)?
      (4) who provides the data?
      (5) how are data transmitted?
      (6) how are data stored?
      (7) who analyzes the data?
      (8) how are data analyzed and how often?
      (9) how often are reports generated?
      (10) to whom are reports disseminated?
      (11) how are reports disseminated?
   d. level of usefulness (users of data and actions taken)
   e. system attributes
      (1) simplicity
      (2) flexibility
      (3) sensitivity
      (4) reliability
      (5) acceptability
      (6) positive predictive value
      (7) representativeness
      (8) timeliness
   f. system resource requirements (direct costs)
      (1) personnel
      (2) other (computer & office equipment, travel, training, mobile phone)
3. Epidemic preparedness and outbreak response
   a. plan of action and coordinating committee
      (1) public health incident command system (PHICS)
      (2) cholera command and control center (C4)
   b. clinical case definitions

c. case mgmt guidelines for communicable diseases with epidemic potential
d. outbreak mgmt protocol
   (1) surveillance definitions
   (2) alert thresholds
   (3) rapid response teams to investigate case reports
   (4) epidemic investigation kits to use
   (5) specimens to collect
   (6) labs to verify diagnosis (including sample sharing for confirmatory testing)
   (7) patients to identify, isolate, and treat (inpatient and outpatient settings)
      (a) isolation areas to organize
      (b) treatments to plan
   (8) contacts to trace and ? quarantine
   (9) hotlines to use for notifiable diseases and investigation of rumor
e. primary and secondary prevention
   (1) infection control protocols
   (2) commodities
      (a) vaccines (eg measles, meningitis)
      (b) drugs (eg prophylactic meds)
      (c) chemicals (eg soap, Ca hypochlorite)
      (d) supplies (eg chlorimetric and colimetric monitors)
      (e) equipment (eg PPE)
f. resource prepositioning (stockpiles, supply chain)
g. information mgmt and crisis communication (media strategy)
   (1) health authorities, WHO
   (2) political authorities
   (3) community leaders and public
      (a) social mobilization
      (b) hygiene promotion and health education
      (c) behavioral change communication (BCC)
h. contingency planning for epidemic consequences
   (1) provision of essential services (lifelines)
   (2) corpse mgmt

4. Health promotion
   a. targeted diseases
      (1) acute epidemic diseases
      (2) chronic diseases – HTN, DM, HIV/TB, asthma
   b. health promotion activities
      (1) community health education
      (2) provider education

5. Health protection (if significant to disaster response)
    a. air quality (eg wildfires, volcanic eruptions)
    b. injury control
    c. occupational health and safety
    d. hazardous materials (eg chemical releases)
    e. disaster risk reduction (eg safe hospitals)
6. Issues summary

B. Health Facilities and Clinical Services

	Fixed Clinics	Health Centers	District Hospitals
1. Quantity			
2. Catchment population			
benchmark	5–10 k	< 50 k	100 k
3. Access to facility			
benchmark	self	self	referral
4. Staffing			
a. quantity (~1/1000 population)			
benchmark	2–5	5–10	variable
b. skill mix			
benchmark	1 HCW	5 HCW, 1 MD	5 MD, 1 surg
5. Caseload (110% of catchment population/d)			
benchmark	1%	1%	
6. Bed capacity (10/10,000 population)			
7. Bed occupancy			
8. Referral load (10% of caseload)			
benchmark	10%	10%	
9. Referral system			
10. Clinical services	OPD, ORS	+ IPD, L&D	+ OR
a. departments/units (verify functioning of expected services)			
(1) clinical			
(a) OPD	+	+	+
(b) IPD	-	+	+
(c) L&D	-	+	+
(d) surgery	-	+/–	+
(e) other			
(2) dispensary	+/–	+	+
(3) diagnostic lab	+/–	+	+
(4) blood bank	-	-	+
(5) radiology	-	-	+
b. special services (verify quality of care)			
(1) child health			
(a) EPI			
(b) IMCI			
(c) child protection			

(2) reproductive health (20% of P_T are F 15–44 yr; 20% (4% of P_T) are pregnant, 20% (4% of P_T) are lactating)
   (a) identify RH lead agency
   (b) prevent and manage consequences of sexual & gender-based violence (SGBV)
      (i) emergency contraception (post rape)
   (c) reduce HIV transmission
      (i) abstain, be faithful, use condoms (ABCs)
      (ii) standard precautions
      (iii) treatment of STIs
      (iv) PMTCT
   (d) safe motherhood—basic & comprehensive emergency OB care
      (i) antenatal care
      (ii) professional midwifery
      (iii) clean delivery
      (iv) essential newborn care
      (v) referral options
   (e) family planning
      (i) general contraception
(3) trauma
   (a) (para)military conflict
   (b) domestic violence
   (c) rape
   (d) motor vehicle trauma
(4) mental health
   (a) adjustment disorders (eg debilitating grief reactions)
   (b) psychiatric disease (eg psychoses, affective disorders) (severe—baseline 2–3% of P_T + 1% increase post-disaster (net 50% increase); mild-mod—baseline 10% of P_T + 5–10% increase post-disaster (net 50–100% increase))
   (c) violence
   (d) drug abuse
(5) chronic diseases (20% of P_T)
   (a) HTN
   (b) DM
   (c) HIV/TB
   (d) asthma
   (e) other

c. standardized case management
   (1) clinical case definitions
   (2) treatment protocols (ORS + Zn, ABX, ACT, IPT, and ITN will save 75% of U5 deaths)

        (3) other clinical protocols (standard precautions, injection safety, medical waste mgmt)
        (4) essential (standard) drugs and rational drug use
            (a) EHKs
            (b) specialty kits
        (5) referral guidelines
        (6) secondary prevention
    d. infection control
        (1) dedicated staff
        (2) hand washing facilities
        (3) stocks of essential supplies (soap, gloves, masks, gowns)
        (4) infection control protocols
        (5) compliance
11. Utilities
    a. power supply
    b. water supply
    c. excreta disposal/septic system
12. Issues summary

C. Human Resources

	Available/10,000 p	Needed (quantity)
1. Basic (not vocationally trained)		
a. traditional birth attendant		
b. community health worker		
c. nurse's aide		
d. other applicable		
2. Mid, High (vocationally trained)		
a. surgical/lab/pharmacy tech		
b. nurse		
c. midwife		
d. pharmacist		
e. doctor		
f. health facility administrator		
g. public health staff (identify)		
h. other applicable		

3. Major areas with staff shortage
4. Reasons for staff shortage (eg security, migration, salary)
5. Issues summary

D. Essential Medical Products and Technologies

1. National standards
    a. essential medicines formulary
    b. standardized equipment per level of care
    c. diagnostic protocols

   d. treatment protocols
2. Procurement of commodities
   NB vaccines & drugs should be on national formulary, from WHO approved manufacturer, and of proven quality
   a. vaccines
   b. drugs
   c. chemicals (eg lab reagents)
   d. diagnostics
   e. supplies (eg chlorine, soap, gloves, masks)
   f. equipment
3. Warehousing
   a. warehouse security
   b. complete storage of commodities in warehouse
   c. arrangements of pallets and shelves
   d. inventory system with stock cards—especially for drugs (SUMA)
   e. documentation of inflows and outflows
   f. central reporting
4. Distribution system (medical logistics)
   a. product availability and price monitoring system
   b. supervision of peripheral facilities
5. Provider training program for rational prescribing
6. Regulatory system
7. Issues summary

E. Health Information Systems

1. Vital
2. Clinical
3. Laboratory
4. Epidemiological
5. Financial
6. Issues summary

F. Health Financing

1. Subsidies
2. Costs, charges, and waivers
3. Provider incentives
4. Issues summary

G. Health Leadership and Governance

	MOH	PHO	DHO
1. Name			
2. Title			
3. Areas/programs of responsibility			
4. Working hours			
5. Communication methods			
6. Stated needs			
7. Organogram with contact list			

8. Issues summary

References

1. UNICEF. Statistical tables. In: *The State of the World's Children*. New York: UNICEF, annual. Available from: http://www.unicef.org/sowc/.
2. WHO. Global Health Indicators. In: *World Health Statistics*. Geneva: World Health Organization, annual. Available from: Global Health Observatory at http://www.who.int/gho/publications/world_health_statistics/en/.
3. US Centers for Disease Control and Prevention. (2001). Updated guidelines for evaluating public health surveillance systems—Recommendations from the Guidelines Working Group. *Morbidity and Mortality Weekly Report, 50*(RR-13):1–35.

Document 1.4
EMERGENCY MANAGEMENT SYSTEM PROFILE

I. EMERGENCY/DISASTER LEGISLATION AND POLICY

A. Statutory Definitions (emergency, disaster, etc)

B. Legal Assignment of Roles and Responsibilities for Disaster Management (National Emergency Response Plan, National MCI Management Plan, Model State Emergency Health Powers Act)

1. Disaster management authority
2. Disaster warning and declaration
3. Disaster plan activation
4. Disaster command and control
5. EOC/ICS stand-up and function
6. Disaster assessment team(s) deployment
7. Essential services provision
8. Resource mobilization and management
    a. technical assistance
    b. material assistance (supply management)
    c. financial assistance
    d. volunteer assistance
    e. coordination of assistance
9. Authorities for drawing extra-budgetary funds in emergency operations
10. Authorities for appeal for external assistance (mutual aid agreements, etc)
11. Public information
12. Contingency planning
13. Field reporting and restrictions

C. Special Emergency Powers (protection of persons)

1. Regulation of professionals (licensing, credentialing, privileging)
2. Civil liability, immunity, and indemnification
3. Protection from harms (workers' compensation)

D. Ad Hoc Advisories and Decrees

1. Law enforcement decrees (border control, curfew, lockdown, etc)
2. Health decrees (quarantine, burial, etc)
3. Immunization campaigns
4. Personnel mobilization
5. Customs procedures (drugs, supplies, equipment)

II. COORDINATION OF AUTHORITIES

A. Lead Agency

1. Roles and responsibilities
2. Locus of control
3. Level and span of authority
4. Full and part-time staff
5. Chain of command
6. Reporting methods
7. Budget
8. Other resources
9. Policy
10. Programs
11. Contingency plans
12. Stated needs
13. Reliability
14. Organogram with contact list

B. Stakeholders

1. Government
   a. central
   b. provincial/state
   c. local
2. Ministries involved in disaster management
   a. civil defense
   b. foreign affairs
   c. communications
   d. transportation
   e. housing
   f. health
   g. hazard-specific agencies (seismology, etc)
3. Emergency services
   a. police
   b. fire
   c. ambulance
   d. hospitals
   e. others
4. Military
5. Private sector
   a. academia
   b. business
   c. community leaders
6. UN agencies & IOs
7. NGOs

C. Mechanism of Coordination

1. Individual disaster preparedness activities
2. Joint disaster preparedness activities
3. MOU with other agencies or institutions
4. Mutual aid agreements
5. National program on disaster preparedness
6. Field-based coordination

III. DISASTER PLANS—GENERIC ALL-HAZARDS

A. Conceptual Framework

1. All hazards approach
   a. hazard-specific contingency plans
2. Comprehensive approach (PPRR)
3. Integrated (all agencies) approach
4. Prepared community
5. Resilient community

B. Incident Management Principles

1. Common terminology
   a. organizational functions
   b. resource descriptions
   c. incident facilities
2. Modular organization
3. Management by objectives
4. Incident action planning
5. Manageable span of control (3–7)
6. Incident facilities and locations
   a. command posts
   b. bases
   c. staging areas
   d. mass casualty triage areas
   e. point of distribution sites
7. Comprehensive resource management
8. Integrated communications
9. Establishment and transfer of command
   a. scope, jurisdiction, authority
   b. standardized briefing at handover
10. Chain of command (orderly line of authority) and unity of command (all individuals have designated supervisor)
11. Unified command (allows agencies with different legal, geographic, and functional authorities to cooperate in multi-agency or multi-jurisdiction environment without compromising individual agency responsibility, authority, or accountability)
12. Accountability (of resources)

13. Dispatch/deployment (only on authorization and request)
14. Information management

C. Disaster Plan Development (national/state/local/institutional)

1. Office(r) in charge of preparedness planning
2. Dedicated budget for preparedness planning
3. Planning scenarios

D. Disaster Plan Components

1. Disaster authorities
2. Disaster warning and declaration
3. Disaster plan activation (levels)
4. Disaster command and control (ICS)
   a. command (responsibility vs authority)
   b. operations
   c. planning
   d. logistics
   e. finance
5. Emergency operations center
   a. command (degree of autonomy)
   b. SOPs
   c. communications (interoperability)
   d. site selection (accessibility)
   e. support services (food, fuel, etc for self-sufficiency)
6. Disaster assessment team(s) deployment
7. Essential services provision (scene operations)
   a. command and control
   b. communications
   c. damage assessment
   d. evacuation
   e. firefighting
   f. law enforcement, safety, and security
   g. emergency health services provision
   h. shelter and mass care
   i. respite care
   j. secondary disaster prevention and hazard mitigation
   k. public information
      (1) information content
      (2) dissemination
      (3) media relations
      (4) special advisories and declarations
         (a) health decrees (quarantine, burial, restrictions, bans, etc)
         (b) immunization campaigns
         (c) personnel mobilization
         (d) drug importation

8. Recovery operations
9. Resource mobilization (see VI)
   a. directory of key personnel
   b. inventory of critical resources
   c. spending authorities

IV. DISASTER PLANS—HAZARD-SPECIFIC ANNEXES

A. Natural Disasters

B. Technological Disasters

C. Conflict and Complex Emergencies

V. DISASTER PLANS—HEALTH SECTOR-SPECIFIC FUNCTIONS (adapted from DHHS [1], [2])

A. Preparedness of Community and Healthcare System

1. Community
   a. determine risks to public health
   b. build community partnerships
   c. foster health-related social networks
   d. coordinate community engagement
2. Healthcare system
   a. develop healthcare coalitions
   b. coordinate healthcare planning within the healthcare system
   c. prioritize essential healthcare assets and services
   d. identify gaps and mitigate them
   e. plan for at-risk groups with special needs
   f. coordinate training of healthcare workers
   g. conduct exercises and evaluation

B. Emergency Operations Coordination

1. Conduct preliminary assessment to determine need for disaster activation
2. Activate public health emergency operations
   a. pre-identified key staff must respond in 60 minutes or less
3. Develop incident response strategy
   a. incident action plan must be produced and approved before the start of the 2nd operational period
4. Manage and sustain the public health response
5. Demobilize and evaluate public health emergency operations

C. Public Health Surveillance/Epidemiological Investigation

1. Conduct public health surveillance and detection
2. Conduct public health and epidemiological investigations
3. Recommend, monitor, and analyze mitigation actions
4. Improve public health/epidemiological investigation systems

D. Public Health Laboratory Testing

1. Manage laboratory activities
2. Perform sample management
3. Conduct testing and analysis for routine and surge capacity
4. Support public health investigations
5. Report results

E. Information Sharing

1. Identify stakeholders to be incorporated into information flow
2. Identify and develop data elements and rules for sharing
3. Exchange information to determine a common operating picture

F. Emergency Public Information and Warning

1. Activate emergency public information system
2. Determine the need for a joint public information system
3. Establish and participate in information system operations
4. Establish avenues for pubic interaction and information exchange
5. Issue public information, alerts, warnings, and notifications

G. Medical Surge

1. Assess the nature and scope of the incident
2. Support activation of medical surge
3. Support jurisdictional medical surge operations
4. Support demobilization of medical surge operations

H. Mass Care

1. Determine mass care needs of the impacted population
2. Determine public health role in mass care operations
3. Coordinate public health, medical, and mental/behavioral health services
4. Monitor mass care population health

I. Medical Countermeasure Dispensing

1. Identify and initiate medical countermeasure dispensing strategies
2. Receive medical countermeasures
3. Activate dispensing modalities
4. Dispense medical countermeasures to identified population
5. Report adverse events

J. Medical Materiel Management and Distribution

1. Activate medical materiel management and distribution
2. Acquire medical materiel

3. Maintain updated inventory management and reporting
4. Establish and maintain security
5. Distribute medical materiel
6. Recover medical materiel and demobilize distribution operations

K. Non-Pharmaceutical Interventions

1. Engage partners and identify factors that impact non-pharmaceutical interventions
2. Determine non-pharmaceutical interventions
   a. personal hygiene
   b. isolation and quarantine
   c. travel advisories and movement restrictions
   d. social distancing
   e. external decontamination
   f. precautionary protective behaviors
3. Implement non-pharmaceutical interventions
4. Monitor non-pharmaceutical interventions

L. Responder Safety and Health

1. Identify responder safety and health risks
2. Identify safety and personal protective needs
3. Coordinate with partners to facilitate risk-specific safety and health training
4. Monitor responder safety and health actions

M. Volunteer Management

1. Notify volunteers needed and discourage those not needed
2. Assemble, organize, and dispatch volunteers
3. Coordinate volunteers
4. Demobilize volunteers

N. Fatality Management

1. Determine role for public health in fatality management
2. Activate public health fatality management operations
3. Assist in the collection and dissemination of antemortem data
4. Participate in survivor mental/behavioral health services
5. Participate in fatality processing and storage operations

O. Community and Healthcare System Recovery

1. Community
   a. monitor health system recovery needs
   b. coordinate community health system recovery operations
   c. implement mitigation steps to limit future damages

2. Healthcare system
   a. develop healthcare system recovery processes
   b. assist implementation of continuity of operations planning

VI. DISASTER PLANS – MEDICAL LOGISTICS

A. Key Personnel Directory

1. Quantity, health discipline, and status (fit for duty, availability full-time, part-time)
2. Emergency mobilization
3. Deployment
   a. concentration point
   b. tasking orders
   c. materiel (clothing, PPE, supplies, equipment)
   d. transport
   e. telecommunications

B. Material Resources Inventory

1. Essential relief items (national list with specs and costs; local REA)
2. Sources
   a. existing supplies of essential relief items
   b. manufacturers/suppliers of essential relief items (local - > national)
   c. donations
3. Warehouses
   a. location
   b. size
   c. prepositioned resources (esp essential drugs, supplies, and EH items)
4. Tracking (SUMA)

C. Transportation Systems (land, sea, air)

1. Availability
2. Capacity
3. Costs
4. Key road entry/exit points
5. Fuel storage and distribution system

D. Telecommunication Systems

1. Country infrastructure
2. Government emergency communications center
   a. technologies
      (1) phone
      (2) fax
      (3) telex

(4) e-mail
(5) ham radio
(6) satellite

b. geographic range
c. legal and technical restrictions on use

3. Disaster preparedness program communications center
4. Disaster management contact information
    a. national government
    b. MOH
    c. academic institutions, private sector
    d. donor organizations
    e. list of organizations operating in country (esp emergency response capacity)
    f. list of reference centers and resource persons with hazard-specific expertise
    g. community preparedness focal points

E. **Evacuation Planning**

1. Triggers
2. Routes
3. Shelters

F. **Program Budget**

1. Regular budget
2. Extra-budgetary (emergency operations)

Reference

1. US Centers for Disease Control and Prevention, Office of Public Health Preparedness and Response. (2011). *Public health preparedness capabilities: national standards for state and local planning*. Available from: www.cdc.gov/phpr/capabilities.
2. US Dept of Health and Human Services, Office of the Assistant Secretary for Preparedness and Response, and US Centers for Disease Control and Prevention, Office of Public Health Preparedness and Response. (2012). *Healthcare preparedness capabilities: national guidance for healthcare system preparedness*. Available from: http://www.phe.gov/preparedness/planning/hpp/pages/default.aspx.

2 Field Assessment

Contents

Overview

This section provides guidance on post-disaster field assessment. Many assessments will occur in the post-disaster health sector. These include assessments of facility damage, medical logistics, health status, nutritional status, needs, hazards, probabilities, vulnerabilities, capabilities, risk, etc. However, numerous problems surround survey team leaders, issues in statistical representativeness, piloting of data gathering instruments, and complicated data management processes.

Generic data collection forms should be standardized for the region and customized by parties to a (sub)national assessment. Such forms may already exist at MOH. If not, forms from external sources may be helpful though modifications may be needed and should be done in collaboration with the MOH. Forms should be simple with standard definitions and minimum essential data sets (MEDS) to avoid overburdening field workers. Field conditions are fluid, data are perishable, and informants are fickle. In collecting field data relevant for decision-making, several cardinal rules apply:

- Quick and dirty is better than slow and clean.
- The whole picture half right is better than half the picture wholly right.

D. A. Bradt, C. M. Drummond, *Pocket Field Guide for Disaster Health Professionals*,
https://doi.org/10.1007/978-3-030-04801-3_2

- General accuracy is more important than statistical precision.
- Limited data are better than exhaustive data.
- Verified data are better than rumored data.
- Early is essential, and late is useless.

In the acute disaster setting, the only data that deserve collection are those that inform urgent field actions. Agencies may wish to collect additional data, but this should be done only if those data inform other critical decisions. Data gathering for academic researchers, report writing for agency donors, or media relations for advocacy groups are distractors early in a relief operation that divert attention from the operational focus of main effort.

This section focuses on 3 main assessment instruments.

- Rapid epidemiological assessment
- Site-specific assessment
- Feeding center assessment

These assessments are supported by background data on:

- Pre-existing indicators
- Population and infrastructure damage
- Sectoral gap identification

Glossary

ABX	antibiotics
ACAPS	Assessment Capacities Project
ACT	artemisinin-based combination therapy
AGR	annual growth rate
AR	attack rate
ARI	acute respiratory infection
BCC	behavioral change communication
BEmONC	basic emergency obstetric and newborn care
CBR	crude birth rate
CBRNE	chemical, biological, radiological, nuclear, explosive
CD	communicable disease; complex disaster
CDC	Centers for Disease Control and Prevention (US)
CEmONC	comprehensive emergency obstetric and newborn care
CERF	Central Emergency Response Fund (managed by OCHA)
CFR	case fatality rate
Cl	chlorine
CMR	crude mortality rate
CTC	community therapeutic care
d	day
DHF	dengue hemorrhagic fever
DHO	district health office
DM	diabetes mellitus
DPT	diphtheria, pertussis, and tetanus combination vaccine
DR	death rate
DRR	disaster risk reduction
D_T	deaths total
E_0	life expectancy at birth
EHK	Emergency Health Kit
EOC	Emergency Operations Center

EPI	Expanded Programme on Immunization
FUO	fever of unknown origin
GAM	global acute malnutrition
GI	gastrointestinal
GIS	geographic information system
GNI	gross national income
GU	genitourinary
h	hour
HB	hepatitis B
HCW	health care worker
HDR	humanitarian daily ration
HeRAMS	Health Resources Availability and Mapping System
HF	hemorrhagic fever
HIS	health information system
HIV	human immunodeficiency virus
HPN	Humanitarian Practice Network
HTN	hypertension
IASC	Inter-Agency Standing Committee
ICS	incident command system
IDP	internally displaced person
IMCI	Integrated Management of Childhood Illness (WHO and UNICEF program)
IMPAC	Integrated Management of Pregnancy and Childbirth (WHO program)
IMR	infant mortality rate
IPC	Integrated Food Security Phase Classification
IPD	inpatient department
IPT	intermittent preventive treatment (of malaria)
IRA	initial rapid assessment
ITN	insecticide treated net
IYCF	infant and young child feeding
L	liter
L&D	labor and delivery
LBW	low birth weight
LDC	less developed country
m	meter
MIRA	multi-cluster initial rapid assessment
mL	milliliter
MMR	maternal mortality ratio
mo	month
MOH	Ministry of Health
MPS	Making Pregnancy Safer (WHO program)
MS	musculoskeletal
MSF	Médecins sans Frontières
MT	metric ton
NCD	non-communicable disease
NFI	non-food item
NGO	non-governmental organization

NTU	nephelometric turbidity units
O50	over 50 yrs of age
OCHA	Office for the Coordination of Humanitarian Affairs (UN)
OHCHR	Office of the High Commissioner for Human Rights (UN)
OPD	outpatient department
ORS	oral rehydration salts/solution
p	after; person
PDA	personal digital assistant
PDNA	post-disaster needs assessment
PEM	protein energy malnutrition
PHC	primary health care
PHO	provincial health office
PMTCT	prevention of mother-to-child transmission
PPE	personal protective equipment
P_T	population total
$P_{T\text{-}pre}$	population total pre-disaster
RH	reproductive health
RUTF	ready-to-use therapeutic food
SAM	severe acute malnutrition
SAR	search and rescue
SEA	sexual exploitation and abuse
SFP	supplementary feeding program
SGBV	sexual and gender-based violence
SPHC	selective primary health care
SRP	strategic response plan
STI	sexually transmitted infection
SUMA	supply management system (devised by WHO)
SWOT	strengths, weaknesses, opportunities, and threats
TFC	therapeutic feeding center
TFP	therapeutic feeding program
TFR	total fertility rate
TOR	terms of reference
U1	under 1 year-old
U5	under 5 year-old
U5MR	under 5 year-old mortality rate
U10	under 10 year-old
UNDAC	UN Disaster Assessment and Coordination
UNDP	UN Development Programme
UNHCR	UN High Commissioner for Refugees
UNICEF	UN Children's Emergency Fund
USAID	US Agency for International Development
VPI	vaccine preventable illness
WB	World Bank
WFP	World Food Programme (UN)
WHO	World Health Organization (UN)
wk	week
yr	year
Zn	zinc

Document 2.1
PRE-EXISTING INDICATORS

A. Population Affected

1. Census (may be simplified as < 5 yr and ≥ 5 yr)

	M	F	Total
a. < 1			
b. 1–4			
c. 5–14			
d. 15–44			
e. ≥45			
f. total			

2. Demography
   a. race, ethnicity, religion
   b. languages
   c. socioeconomic status
   d. urban vs rural
   e. average family/household size

B. Settlements

1. Overall size of affected area
2. Locations
   a. community size, geographic separation
   b. access to transportation hubs and communication links
3. Population mobility
4. Community density
   a. geographic separation of families within the settlement
5. Shelter type and quality
6. Hazard exposure (eg upcoming seasonal natural hazards)
7. Equality/discrimination within the community
8. Conflict within the community
9. Emergency preparedness
10. Known coping mechanisms

C. Access to Essential Services (see UNICEF [1], WHO [2])

1. Public utilities (infrastructure)
   a. % population with access to improved water
   b. % population with access to improved sanitation
   c. % population with electricity
   d. % population with telephones/television

2. Health services
   a. skilled health care workers (all)/10,000 p (23)
   b. physicians/10,000 p (0.2)
   c. nurses/10,000 p (1)
   d. midwives/10,000 p (1)
   e. community health workers/10,000 p (10)
   f. % population with provider coverage (100%)
   g. consultations/p/yr (1)
   h. % pregnancies receiving antenatal care (100%)
   i. % deliveries attended by trained staff (90%)
   j. % immunization rates—measles vac in 1 y/o (90%)
   k. hospital beds/10,000 p (10)
   l. health facilities with BEmONC, CEmONC/500,000 p (4, 1)
   m. admissions/10,000 p
3. Underserved areas (by location and type of service)

D. Health Status (see UNICEF[1], WHO[2])

1. Mortality and other rates
   a. CBR (10–50)
   b. CMR (5–25)
   c. AGR (%)
   d. IMR (3–200)
   e. U5MR (3–300)
   f. MMR (5–2,100)
   g. E0 at birth M/F/T (40–85)
   h. TFR (2–8)
2. Nutritional status
   a. caloric intake/p/d (2,100 kcal)
   b. % infants with low birth weight (LBW) (7% with <2.5 kg)
   c. % U5 with growth faltering (30%)
   d. % U5 with global acute malnutrition (GAM) (10%)
   e. % with micronutrient deficiencies (vitamins A-D; Fe, I)
   f. % of food supply from international food assistance (WFP, NGOs)
3. Endemic diseases
   a. HIV prevalence
   b. TB prevalence
   c. malaria incidence
   d. other major diseases
4. Health beliefs and traditions
5. Sources of care
6. Referral system

E. Macroeconomic Status (see UNICEF [1], UNDP [3], WB [4])

1. Labor force occupations
   a. agriculture
   b. pastoralism
   c. industry
   d. services
2. Unemployment rate
3. GNI per capita ($US)
4. Inflation rate
5. % population in extreme poverty (<$1.90/d income)
6. Gini index (Gini coefficient × 100 expressed as %) (0–100)
7. general government health expenditures as % of general govt total expenditure (1–25)
8. Current health expenditures as % of GDP (2.5–16)
9. Current health expenditures per capita ($30–10,000)

F. Educational Status (see UNICEF [1])

1. Adult literacy rate
2. Female literacy rate

G. Developmental Status (see UNDP [3])

1. Human development index
2. Fragile states typology (USAID)
   a. post-conflict transition
   b. early recovery
   c. arrested development
   d. deterioration
3. Risk of humanitarian crisis and disaster (see Inform Index [5])

References

1. UNICEF. Statistical Tables. In *The State of the World's Children*. New York: UNICEF, annual. Available from http://www.unicef.org/sowc/.
2. WHO. Global Health Indicators. In *World Health Statistics*. Geneva: World Health Organization, annual. Available from Global Health Observatory at http://www.who.int/gho/publications/world_health_statistics/en/.
3. United Nations Development Programme. Statistical Annex. In: *Human Development Reports*. New York: UNDP, annual. Available from http://www.hdr.undp.org/en.
4. World Bank. *World Development Indicators*. Washington, DC: World Bank, annual. Available from http://wdi.worldbank.org/tables.
5. Marin-Ferrer M, Vernaccini L, and Poljansek K. Index for Risk Management INFORM Concept and Methodology Report, 2017, EUR 28655 EN, https://doi.org/10.2760/094023.

Document 2.2
RAPID EPIDEMIOLOGICAL ASSESSMENT

Date

I. INTRODUCTION (copy A-B to Exec Summary)

A. Hazard History Abridged

B. Current Disaster

1. When
2. Who/what
3. Where/extent
4. Hazard magnitude/concentration/exposure time
5. Mechanism of impact
6. Secondary disaster (eg fire after earthquake, landslide after cyclone)
7. Area affected
8. Population affected

C. Immediate Response of Host Government Authorities

1. Disaster declaration
2. Disaster plan activation
3. Disaster command and control
4. Emergency operations center
5. Disaster assessment team(s)

D. Your Mission

1. Request by host authorities (person, position)
2. Acceptance by your organization (person, position)
3. Objectives (per TOR, examples below)
   a. assess disaster impact
   b. identify unmet needs in the health sector
   c. advise MOH/PHO/DHO of disaster impact and unmet needs
   d. recommend actions to prevent and/or control communicable diseases of epidemic potential
   e. assist with adaptation of normative technical best practices for local implementation
   f. plan goals, objectives, and projects for follow-up action by your agency
   g. provide on-site clinical care (substitution)
   h. provide on-site health sector coordination (substitution)
   i. monitor progress in disaster relief, rehabilitation, and recovery

j. advocate with local and international donors for support of unmet needs of vulnerable populations
k. contribute to local/regional health clusters or working groups as appropriate

II. SOURCES AND METHODS

A. Assessment Team Composition

B. Assessment Area and Dates

C. Information Sources and Assessment Methods

1. Review of secondary source data
   a. records and reports
   b. surveys and surveillance
   c. testimonies
   d. photographs and maps
2. Primary data gathered in structured and unstructured formats
   a. direct observation (site visits and transect walks)
   b. key informant interviews (institutions, field sites, and/or households)
   c. convenience sampling of target population (eg community leaders, HCWs, members of vulnerable groups)
   d. focus (community) group discussions

D. Logistics of Assessment Team

E. Constraints

1. Security
2. Access
3. Transport
4. Telecommunications
5. Truth telling

III. PRE-EXISTING INDICATORS (summarize Doc 2.1)

IV. DISASTER IMPACT

A. Area Affected (focus on most affected)
1. Geographic extent
2. Political jurisdictions (eg states, districts)

B. Population Affected (focus on most affected; see Doc 2.5)

1. Population morbidity & mortality
   a. dead (rates generally not used for deaths from a single discrete event)
   b. injured
      (1) hospital admissions
         (a) evacuated
      (2) outpatients
   c. missing or unaccounted

2. Population undisplaced but crisis-affected
   a. accessible
   b. inaccessible/isolated
   c. host families (# or % of catchment population)
   d. total needing humanitarian assistance
3. Population displaced from usual homes

	IDPs	refugees
a. in organized camps or dispersed in camp-like settings		
b. in group accommodation apart from above		
c. in host families or individual accommodation		
d. new arrivals (specify time period)		
e. resettled		
f. total needing humanitarian assistance		

4. Surviving vulnerable groups

	IDPs	refugees
a. U5		
b. malnourished		
c. orphaned		
d. abandoned		
e. pregnant		
f. lactating		
g. disabled		
h. elderly		
i. total needing humanitarian assistance		

C. Damage Assessment (focus on most affected area; see Doc 2.5)

1. Material losses	destroyed	heavy damage	light damage
a. homes			
b. commercial buildings			
c. industrial buildings			
(1) hazmat facilities			
d. public buildings			
(1) govt administration			
(2) hospitals			
(3) health centers			
(4) schools			
(5) community shelters			
(6) police stations			
(7) fire stations			

e. infrastructure/lifelines	disrupted (%)	restored (%)
(1) telecommunications		
(a) landlines		
(b) mobiles		

        (c) satellite phones
        (d) radio net
        (e) internet
    (2) transportation network
        (a) roads
        (b) railroads
        (c) airports
        (d) seaports
    (3) utilities
        (a) electrical power supply
        (b) water supply
        (c) waste disposal

2. Financial impact (PDNA)
   a. direct damages
   b. indirect losses
   c. impact on major sources of income (eg agriculture, industry)

D. Secondary Disasters and Threats

1. Secondary phenomena (eg floods after storms)
2. Hazard recurrence
3. Weather complications and predictions
4. Epidemics
5. CBRNE consequences
6. Areas of concern (eg flooding → gastroenteritis, hepatitis, leptospirosis, dengue, malaria, vipers)

E. Disaster Impact Summary

V. CURRENT EPIDEMIOLOGICAL INDICATORS

A. Epidemiology

1. Mortality
   a. total deaths, excess mortality
   b. proportional mortality
      (1) cause-specific proportion of D_T (diarrhea, measles have each caused up to 40% of D_T in acute disasters)
      (2) D_T/P_T % (if $D_T \geq 1\%$ of P_T)
   c. death rates & trends
      (1) crude (<1/10,000/d; >2 is critical)
      (2) age-specific eg 0–5 DR (<2/10,000/d; >4 is critical) (often 50% of D_T)
      (3) disease-specific (uncommonly used)
      (4) excess (crisis death rate – baseline death rate)

d. case-fatality ratios
   (1) diarrhea (cholera 2–50%, dysentery 2–20%; target is CFR < 1%)
   (2) ARI (pneumonia 2–20%)
   (3) malaria
   (4) measles (2–30%)
   (5) malnutrition (25–50% in SAM; associated with 50% of U5 deaths)
   (6) trauma (20% of civilian injured in acute military conflict)

2. Morbidity
   a. total cases
   b. proportional morbidity
      (1) acute disease (epi estimates underlying early versions of EHK)
         (a) adult presentations (1 adult obtains ~4 consults/yr; 5,000 adults obtain ~5,000 consults/3 mo) % adults presenting with: GI 25%, ARI 20%, MS 15%, GU 15%, malaria 10%, trauma 5%, anemia 5%, ocular 5%
         (b) pedes (1 child obtains ~5 consults/yr; 5,000 children obtain ~6,500 consults/3 mo) % pedes presenting with: GI 30%, ARI 30%, worms 20%, malaria 15%, trauma 10%, anemia 10%, ocular 10%, otic 5%
      (2) chronic disease (20% of P_T)
   c. incidence rates & trends
      (1) presentation rate/d (1% baseline – 10% in CDs)
      (2) age-specific (high risk = U5, O50)
      (3) disease-specific (DART MMMM)
         (a) **d**iarrhea (AR 50%/mo in U5 excluding below)
            (i) dysentery (AR 5–30% over 1–3 mo in P_T)
            (ii) cholera (AR 1–5% over 1–4 mo in P_T)
         (b) **AR**I (AR 50%/mo in U5 esp in cold weather)
         (c) **m**alaria (AR 50%/mo in P_T non-immune; 2%/mo in P_T immune (WHO))
            holo-endemic—intense transmission year-round (Congo) (6–10 infections/child/yr; mortality highest in U5 & pregnant F)
            hyper-endemic—intense transmission seasonally (W. Afr) (4–6 infections/child/yr; mortality across all ages)
            hypo-endemic—low transmission year-round (Thai-Burma) (1 infection/person/yr; mortality across all ages)

(d) **m**easles (AR 10%/epidemic in U12 non-immunized; 10–75% of cases with complications depending on health status)
(e) **m**alnutrition
  (i) macro (PEM 10% with $Z < -2$, 1% with $Z < -3$)
  (ii) micro (vitamins A–D; Fe, I)
(f) **t**rauma
  (i) (para)military conflict
  (ii) rape
  (iii) domestic violence
  (iv) motor vehicle trauma
(g) **m**ental health
  (i) adjustment disorders (debilitating grief reactions)
  (ii) psychiatric disease (eg psychoses, affective disorders) (severe—baseline 2–3% of P_T severe + 1% increase post-disaster (net 50% increase); mild-mod—baseline 10% of P_T + 5–10% increase post-disaster (net 50–100% increase))
  (iii) violence
  (iv) drug abuse

B. Outbreaks and Epidemics

1. Recent or ongoing
   a. etiology
   b. date of first case(s)
   c. location
   d. number of cases or attack rate
   e. consequences or current status
2. Potential (see REA IV D 6)
   a. wide geographic relevance
      (1) measles
      (2) cholera (dehydrating diarrhea)
      (3) shigella (bloody diarrhea)
      (4) meningococcus (meningitis)
      (5) hepatitis A, E (acute jaundice syndrome)
      (6) influenza
      (7) other
   b. specific geographic relevance
      (1) malaria
      (2) dengue
      (3) viral hemorrhagic fevers (eg yellow fever, lassa fever, dengue HF)
      (4) typhoid (FUO)
      (5) leishmaniasis
      (6) rare but significant (polio, typhus, plague)
      (7) vectors

(8) vermin
(9) vipers
c. specific age groups
(1) polio (acute flaccid paralysis)
(2) neonatal tetanus

C. Epidemiological Summary

VI. HEALTH SECTOR FUNCTIONAL STATUS

A. Public Health Services (focus on service disruptions, adequacy)

1. Disease prevention
a. primary prevention
(1) vaccine coverage rates for major antigens (EPI coverage rate > 90%)
(a) measles
(b) DPT
(2) vaccine stocks

	quantity available	location
(a) measles		
(b) DPT		
(c) polio		
(d) hepatitis B		
(e) other		

(3) cold chain adequacy
(4) staff adequacy
(5) transport adequacy
(6) most recent campaign in area
(a) location
(b) dates
(c) organizer
(d) coverage
(7) other VPIs of epidemic potential
b. communicable disease control programs

	Y / N	issues
(1) diarrhea		
(2) ARI		
(3) malaria		
(4) HIV		
(5) TB		
(6) other		

2. Epidemiological surveillance system (CDC[1])
a. system objectives
(1) case detection (CDs, NCDs eg malnutrition)
(2) outbreak detection
(3) epidemic forecasting
(4) trend monitoring

(5) priority setting
(6) workload estimation
(7) resource targeting & health program activity
(8) intervention evaluation

b. health events/indicator conditions and case definitions
c. system components and flow chart of operations
(1) what is the population under surveillance?
(2) what is the time period of data collection?
(3) what data are collected (standardized forms)?
(4) who provides the data?
(5) how are data transmitted?
(6) how are data stored?
(7) who analyzes the data?
(8) how are data analyzed and how often?
(9) how often are reports generated?
(10) to whom are reports disseminated?
(11) how are reports disseminated?

d. level of usefulness (users of data and actions taken)
e. system attributes
(1) simplicity
(2) flexibility
(3) sensitivity
(4) reliability
(5) acceptability
(6) positive predictive value
(7) representativeness
(8) timeliness

f. system resource requirements (direct costs)
(1) personnel
(2) other (computer & office equipment, travel, training, mobile phone)

3. Epidemic preparedness and response
a. plan of action and coordinating committee
(1) public health incident command system (PHICS)
(2) cholera command and control center (C4)

b. clinical case definitions
c. case mgmt guidelines for communicable diseases with epidemic potential
d. outbreak mgmt protocol
(1) surveillance definitions
(2) alert thresholds
(3) rapid response teams to investigate case reports
(4) epidemic investigation kits to use
(5) specimens to collect
(6) labs to verify diagnosis (including sample sharing for confirmatory testing)

- (7) patients to identify, isolate, and treat (inpatient and out-patient settings)
  - (a) isolation areas to organize
  - (b) standardized case management to plan
- (8) contacts to trace and ? quarantine
- (9) hotlines to use for notifiable diseases and rumor investigation

e. primary and secondary prevention
- (1) infection control protocols
- (2) commodities
  - (a) vaccines (eg measles, meningitis)
  - (b) drugs (eg prophylactic meds)
  - (c) chemicals (eg soap, Ca hypochlorite)
  - (d) supplies (eg chlorimetric and colimetric monitors)
  - (e) equipment (eg PPE)

f. resource prepositioning (stockpiles, supply chain)

g. information mgmt and crisis communication (media strategy)
- (1) health authorities, WHO
- (2) political authorities
- (3) community leaders and public
  - (a) social mobilization
  - (b) hygiene promotion and health education
  - (c) behavioral change communication (BCC)

h. contingency planning for epidemic consequences
- (1) provision of essential services (lifelines)
- (2) corpse mgmt

4. Health promotion
   a. targeted diseases
      - (1) acute epidemic diseases
      - (2) chronic diseases—HTN, DM, HIV/TB, asthma
   b. health promotion activities
      - (1) community health education
      - (2) provider education
5. Health protection (if significant to disaster response)
   a. air quality (eg wildfires, volcanic eruptions)
   b. injury control
   c. occupational health and safety
   d. hazardous materials (eg chemical releases)
   e. disaster risk reduction (eg safe hospitals)
6. Issues summary

B. Health Facilities and Clinical Services (focus on service disruptions, adequacy; see Document 2.5)

	Fixed Clinics	Health Centers	District Hospitals

1. Quantity
2. Catchment population
3. Access to facility
4. Staffing
   a. quantity (~1/1000 population)
   b. skill mix
5. Caseload (1–10% of catchment population/d)
6. Bed capacity (10/10,000 population)
7. Bed occupancy
8. Referral load (10% of caseload)
9. Referral system
10. Clinical services
    a. departments/units (verify functioning of expected services)
       (1) clinical
          (a) OPD
          (b) IPD
          (c) L&D
          (d) surgery
          (e) other
       (2) dispensary
       (3) diagnostic lab
       (4) blood bank
       (5) radiology
    b. special services (verify quality of care)
       (1) child health
          (a) Expanded Programme on Immunization (EPI)
          (b) Integrated Management of Childhood Illness (IMCI)
          (c) child protection
       (2) reproductive health (20% of P_T are F 15–44 yr; 20% (4% of P_T) are pregnant, 20% (4% of P_T) are lactating)
          (a) identify RH lead agency
          (b) prevent and manage consequences of SGBV (15–20% lifetime incidence in SSA)
             (i) acute trauma care
             (ii) emergency contraception (post-rape)
             (iii) post-exposure prophylaxis
             (iv) psyc follow-up

- (c) reduce HIV transmission
  - (i) abstain, be faithful, use condoms (ABCs)
  - (ii) standard precautions
  - (iii) treatment of STIs
  - (iv) PMTCT
- (d) safe motherhood—basic & comprehensive emergency OB care
  - (i) antenatal care
  - (ii) professional midwifery
  - (iii) clean delivery
  - (iv) essential newborn care
  - (v) referral options
- (e) family planning
  - (i) general contraception

(3) trauma
- (a) (para)military conflict
- (b) rape
- (c) domestic violence
- (d) motor vehicle trauma

(4) mental health
- (a) adjustment disorders (eg debilitating grief reactions)
- (b) psychiatric disease (eg psychoses, affective, anxiety disorders) (severe—baseline 2–3% of P_T + 1% increase post-disaster = net 50% increase; mild-mod—baseline 10% of P_T + 5–10% increase post-disaster = net 100% increase)
- (c) violence
- (d) drug abuse

(5) chronic diseases (20% of P_T)
- (a) HTN
- (b) DM
- (c) HIV/TB
- (d) asthma
- (e) other

c. standardized case management
- (1) clinical case definitions
- (2) treatment protocols (ORS+Zn, ABX, ACT, IPT, and ITN will save 75% of U5 deaths)
- (3) other clinical protocols
  - (a) standard precautions
  - (b) injection safety
  - (c) medical waste mgmt

    (4) essential (standard) drugs and rational drug use
        (a) EHKs
        (b) specialty kits
    (5) referral guidelines
    (6) secondary prevention
  d. infection control
    (1) dedicated staff
    (2) hand washing facilities
    (3) stocks of essential supplies (soap, gloves, masks, gowns)
    (4) infection control protocols (medical waste mgmt, safe transfusion)
    (5) compliance

11. Utilities
    a. power supply
    b. water supply
    c. excreta disposal/septic system
12. Issues summary

C. Human Resources (focus on catchment area of interest)

Available/10,000 p   Needed (quantity)

1. Basic (not vocationally trained)
    a. traditional birth attendant
    b. community health worker
    c. nurse's aide
    d. other applicable
2. Mid, High (vocationally trained)
    a. surgical/lab/pharmacy tech
    b. nurse
    c. midwife
    d. pharmacist
    e. doctor
    f. health facility administrator
    g. public health staff (identify)
    h. other applicable
3. Major areas with staff shortage
4. Reasons for staff shortage (eg security, migration, salary)
5. Issues summary

D. Essential Medical Products and Technologies (medical logistics)

1. National standards
    a. essential medicines formulary
    b. standardized equipment per level of care
    c. diagnostic protocols
    d. treatment protocols

2. Procurement of commodities
   NB vaccines & drugs should be on national formulary, from WHO approved manufacturer, and of proven quality
   a. vaccines
   b. drugs
   c. chemicals (eg lab reagents)
   d. diagnostics
   e. supplies (eg chlorine, soap, gloves, masks)
   f. equipment
3. Warehousing
   a. warehouse security
   b. complete storage of commodities in warehouse
   c. arrangements of pallets and shelves
   d. inventory system with stock cards—especially for drugs (SUMA)
   e. documentation of inflows and outflows
   f. central reporting
4. Distribution system
   a. product availability and price monitoring system
   b. supervision of peripheral facilities
5. Provider training program for rational prescribing
6. Regulatory system
7. Issues summary

E. Health Information Systems

1. Vital
2. Clinical
3. Laboratory
4. Epidemiological
5. Financial
6. Issues summary

F. Health Financing (disaster-specific)

1. Subsidies
2. Costs, charges, and waivers
3. Provider incentives
4. Issues summary

G. Health Leadership and Governance

	MOH	PHO	DHO
1. Name			
2. Title			
3. Areas/programs of responsibility			
4. Working hours			
5. Communication methods			
6. Stated needs			

7. Organogram with contact list
8. Issues summary

H. **Health Sector Functional Status Summary**

VII. OTHER SECTORS

A. Security

1. Disruption of public services
   a. telecommunications
   b. transportation
   c. fuel supplies
   d. public utilities
   e. refuse collection
   f. medical care
   g. education
2. Breakdown of law and order
   a. looting
   b. black markets
   c. riots and demonstrations
   d. road closures
   e. convoy procedures
3. Military/militia/armed opposition group attacks
   a. major civilian population centers
   b. humanitarian staff
   c. health facilities
   d. relief convoys
   e. relief supplies (in transit or in warehouse)
4. Commercial shutdown
5. Discredited government (lies, corruption, repression)
6. Military command and control
7. Frequent, widespread, or systematic armed violence
8. Incidents (impair access)
   NB access limited by weather, poor infrastructure, denial of permission to move, extortion, as well as overt security incidents
   a. crimes (International Criminal Court Rome Statute) (Article 5)
      (1) genocide (Article 6)
      acts committed with intent to destroy, in whole or in part, a national, ethnic, racial, or religious group
      (2) crimes against humanity (Article 7)
      acts committed as part of a widespread or systematic attack against any civilian population, with knowledge of the attack
      (3) war crimes (Article 8)
         (a) grave breaches of the Geneva Conventions of 12 Aug 1949

(b) serious violations of laws and customs applicable in international armed conflict
(c) serious violations of common article 3 applicable in non-international armed conflict (acts vs persons taking no active part in the hostilities, including armed forces placed hors de combat by sickness, wounds, detention, or other cause)
(d) non-applicability of (c) to internal disturbances (riots, sporadic violence, etc)
(e) other serious violations of laws and customs applicable in non-international armed conflict (// 3b above)

(4) crimes of aggression (provision to be adopted)

b. other incidents
(1) type
(a) bombing and shelling
(b) landmines
(c) improvised explosive devices (IED)
(d) unexploded ordnance (UXO)
(e) sniping
(f) chemical, biological, radiological (CBR) weapons
(g) attacks on critical facilities
(2) perpetrators
(a) law enforcement (interior ministries, police)
(b) host country military & paramilitary groups
(c) rebel groups
(d) armed extremists
(e) armed gangs
(f) street thugs

9. Displacement (IDPs, refugees)
a. reason
b. reception/registration at new site
10. Fears
a. anniversary dates of violence
b. fears of national staff
c. fears in the community
d. rumors of community violence
e. rumors about activities of your agency
11. Issues summary

B. Protection (who, where, from what)

1. Security incidents (per REA VII A)
2. Harmful traditional practices
a. traditional tattoo centers
b. female genital cutting
c. gender-based violence

   d. early marriage
   e. forced marriage
   f. polygamy
   g. wife disinheritance
3. Illegal commercial practices
   a. abduction
   b. trafficking (people, commodities, drugs)
   c. prostitution
   d. child labor with exposure to health and safety risks
4. Non-commercial exploitative/abusive practices
   a. recruitment into armed forces
   b. sexual abuse
   c. child abuse
   d. spousal abuse
5. Issues summary

C. Safety (for all parties to relief operation)

1. Environmental hazards (eg natural hazards, falling debris)
2. Street hazards (eg ground debris, vehicle traffic)
3. Buildings (eg fire safety, structural integrity)
4. Vehicles (eg seatbelts, road worthiness)
5. Hazard mitigation activities
6. Issues summary

D. Search and Rescue (if relevant to relief operation)

1. Persons rescued
2. Areas of activity
3. Anticipated duration of SAR phase of relief operations
4. Issues summary

E. Logistics (esp for relief agencies)

1. Telecommunications
   a. landlines
   b. mobile phones
   c. satellite phones
   d. radio net
   e. internet
2. Transportation, fuel
   a. type
   b. availability
   c. cost
3. Issues summary

F. Environment

1. Climate and weather (exacerbations from seasonal weather, El Nino, climate change)
   a. temperature (heat load)
   b. precipitation
      (1) water storage status
      (2) drought-related restrictions
   c. wind, storms
2. Topography (altitude, terrain, natural hazards)
3. Edaphic factors (soil type, surface water presence, rain water drainage, flora, fauna eg vermin, snakes, infestations)
4. Impacts
   a. site-specific impacts (if focal, give details; if widespread, highlight major aspects)
      (1) present owner
      (2) original use
      (3) overall area (45 m^2/p)
      (4) road access
      (5) water access & drainage (1–6% slope—rise over run)
      (6) site hazards (eg ordnance, toxic waste)
      (7) hazard mitigation feasibility
   b. agriculture impacts
      (1) cropping cycle
      (2) planting status, seed supplies, water supplies
      (3) harvest status
      (4) market availability of produce
      (5) current prices
   c. livestock impacts
      (1) animal nutrition status
      (2) stock rearing
      (3) stock selling
      (4) market availability of animals
      (5) current prices
   d. livelihood impacts
      (1) farmers
      (2) pastoralists
      (3) manufacturers
   e. clinical impacts (particularly where relevant to program service delivery and beneficiary morbidity)
      (1) vectors
      (2) diseases
5. Issues summary

G. Environmental Health

1. Water
   a. sources available & outputs (in order of preference)
      (1) aquifers (deep preferred to shallow)
         (a) wells
         (b) handpumps
         (c) boreholes
      (2) surface water (flowing preferred to still)
         (a) still
         (b) flowing
      (3) fixed storage tanks & bladders
      (4) trucks
      (5) other
   b. access (250 p/water point, <500 m from housing)
   c. distribution/collection method
   d. queue time (< 15′)
   e. quantity (5 L/p/d initially → 15–20 L/p/d after 60 d)
   f. quality
      (1) sources of contamination
         (a) open storage containers
         (b) excreta (latrines, septic tanks)
         (c) dumpsites
         (d) chemical storage facilities (eg fuel depots)
      (2) purification method (at source & end user levels)
      (3) water testing method & results
         (a) 0 coliforms/dL
         (b) 0.05 mg/dL free Cl
         (c) <5 NTU (nephelometric turbidity units) (if hand is visible immersed in water, NTU <5)
2. Sanitation
   NB describe site cleanliness, types of waste, magnitude of problem, collection methods & frequency, disposal methods & site, special issues (eg waste separation) for:
   a. excreta (50-100 p/latrine initially → 20 p/latrine after 60 d, 30 m from housing, 100 m from H_2O)
   b. household waste
      (1) garbage
      (2) sullage
   c. solid waste
   d. medical waste
      (1) sharps
      (2) biologics (eg placentas)
      (3) paper/plastic, dressings, bandages
   e. corpses
   f. dead animals

3. Food
   NB describe overall food security in integrated phase classification (IPC) terms with attention to following major dimensions
   a. availability/adequacy
      (1) quantity (2,100 kcal/p/d min with 10–12% from protein, 17% from fat, plus micronutrients from fresh or fortified foods)
      (2) variety
      (3) market proximity to settlements
   b. access (purchasing ability)
   c. utilization
      (1) food hygiene
      (2) cooking
         (a) equipment availability
         (b) fuel type & availability
         (c) preparation—family vs communal
   d. market stability and resilience
      (1) inflation
      (2) exchange rates
      (3) market performance
         (a) price seasonality
         (b) price volatility
   e. altered livelihood and coping strategies
      (1) livestock sales
      (2) firewood & charcoal sales
      (3) self-employment
      (4) labor migration
      (5) decreased consumption of preferred foods (skipping meals)
      (6) increased consumption of wild foods
      (7) gifts & remittances
      (8) school truancy
      (9) commercial sex work
      (10) organized crime
   f. distributions and targeted feedings (IPC 3+, if U5 GAM > 10%)
      (1) blanket supplementary feeding program (SFP)
      (2) targeted supplementary feeding program
      (3) community therapeutic care (CTC)
      (4) therapeutic feeding program (TFP)
4. Shelter and settlements
   a. shelter
      (1) building materials, construction techniques (eg prefab), and quality
      (2) covered space (3.5 m^2/p; 2 m between shelters)
      (3) adequacy of weather protection
      (4) evidence of damages

b. settlements (build environment)
   (1) locations
   (2) security and safety
   (3) hazard risks (eg fire in camps)
   (4) emergency/contingency planning for risks
   (5) access to communication links, transportation hubs
   (6) community density (p/km^2)
   (7) community leaders identified

5. Emergency relief supplies (non food items)
   a. plastic sheeting
   b. blankets
   c. jerry cans
   d. cooking utensils
   e. hygiene kits
   f. mats
   g. ITN
6. Vector/vermin/vipers, reservoirs
   NB describe type of vectors, magnitude of presence, disease risks, control methods, special issues (eg breeding sites, reservoir management)
   a. mosquitoes
   b. rodents
   c. other
7. Public utilities
   a. power supply
   b. water supply
   c. waste disposal/septic system
8. Issues summary

VIII. RESPONSE OF DOMESTIC AUTHORITIES

A. Disaster Management Mechanism

1. Disaster management authority
2. Disaster warning and declaration
3. Disaster plan activation
4. Disaster command and control
5. EOC/ICS stand-up and function
6. Disaster assessment team(s) deployment
7. Essential services provision
8. Resource mobilization and management
   a. technical assistance
   b. material assistance (supply management)
   c. financial assistance
   d. volunteer assistance
   e. coordination of assistance
9. Domestic donations
10. International appeals (stated needs of health authorities)

11. Public information (press releases, websites)
12. Contingency planning
13. Field reporting and restrictions

B. Emergency Protection Powers in Disasters (model legislation)

1. Regulation of professionals—licensing, credentialing, privileging
2. Immunity, indemnification, and civil liability of providers
3. Protection of workers from harm—exposure limits, compensation

C. Advisories and Decrees

1. Law enforcement decrees (emergency, border control, curfew, etc)
2. Health decrees (quarantine, burial, etc)
3. Immunization campaigns
4. Personnel mobilization
5. Customs procedures (drugs, supplies, equipment)

D. Issues Summary

IX. RESPONSE OF INTERNATIONAL COMMUNITY

A. Coordination of International Assistance

1. HCT
2. UNDAC
3. HC
4. Cluster system
   a. health cluster

B. Intervenors

1. Stakeholder analysis (brief SWOT analysis)
   a. GOs
   b. UN
   c. IOs
   d. NGOs
2. Geographic areas of activity
3. Domains of activity

C. Multi-party Assessments

1. Types
   a. (M)IRA
   b. HeRAMS
   c. HIS
2. Gaps—unmet needs (see Tools 3.T3a, 3.T3b)
3. Beneficiary identification

D. International Appeals (OCHA Financial Tracking Service)

1. Flash
2. CERF
3. SRP

E. Issues Summary

1. [Needs – (Coping Strategy + Assistance) = Unmet Needs]

X. RESPONSE OF REPORTING AGENCY (delete if assessment is multi-party or single purpose undertaking without operational follow-up)

A. Assessment Activities Undertaken

B. Assistance Projects/Activities Undertaken (range of options below)

1. Reallocation of existing local & national resources
2. Revision/refinement of present (medical) practices
   a. use of essential drugs
   b. use of standardized case management
   c. elimination of dated practices
3. Financial assistance (critical funding)
4. Technical assistance (critical skills)
   a. complement donated goods
   b. support appropriate technology
   c. develop information systems
5. Material assistance (critical goods)
   a. essential drugs and vaccines
   b. consumable supplies
   c. other stated needs of health authorities
6. Provision of direct services (substitution)
7. Integration of programming
8. Coordination of external assistance
9. Capacity building of host authorities
10. Civil society partnership and support
    a. organize community leaders
    b. encourage gender mainstreaming
    c. encourage privatization
    d. discourage entitlements
11. Advocacy
12. Transition to early recovery
13. Monitoring and evaluation
    a. remote management system if needed
    b. risk management system to prevent and detect waste, fraud, and abuse

XI. OPERATIONAL CONSTRAINTS

- **A. Security**
- **B. Political/Administrative**
- **C. Logistical**
- **D. Technical**
- **E. Economic**
- **F. Developmental**

XII. REA PRINCIPAL FINDINGS AND ANALYSIS (copy to Exec Sum; list major findings from section summaries; emphasize summaries bolded below as most relevant to health sector; delete headings if simpler to serially list findings; use phrases, not sentences)

- **A. Disaster Impact Summary** (see REA IV E)
- **B. Epidemiological Summary** (see REA V C)
- **C. Health Sector Functional Status Summary** (see REA VI H)
- **D.** Security, Protection, and Safety (see REA VII A,B,C)
- **E.** Search and Rescue (see REA VII D)
- **F.** Logistics (see REA VII E)
- **G.** Environment (see REA VII F)
- **H. Environmental Health** (see REA VII G)
- **I. Stated Needs of Health Authorities** (see REA VIII A10)
- **J. Major Gaps** (see REA IX E)
- **K. Operational Constraints** (see REA XI)
- **L.** Duration of Emergency Phase (see REA VIII C1)
- **M.** Future Risk Factors and Scenario Forecasting (see REA IV D)

Reference

1. US Centers for Disease Control and Prevention. (2001). Updated guidelines for evaluating public health surveillance systems—Recommendations from the Guidelines Working Group. *Morbidity and Mortality Weekly Report, 50*(RR-13):1–35.

Document 2.3
SITE-SPECIFIC ASSESSMENT

Date ______			Assessor ______		
Site Name ______			Informant #1 ______		
Location—GPS/landmark ______			Informant #2 ______		
Population	registration Y N	total pop ______		# households	______
	U1 ______ (5%)	women (15-44)	______ (20%)	arrivals/wk	______
	U5 ______ (20%)	men (15-44)	______ (10%)	departures/wk	______
	5-14 ______ (35%)	45+	______ (15%)	typical livelihood	______
	vulnerable groups ______				
Security	Officer in Charge ______		Camp Leader ______		
Indicators	incidents at site Y N	type (murder, rape, assault) ______			
Issues	______				
Site Mgmt	Lead Agency ______	Contact ______		Ph/Fax ______	
Indicators	original site use ______	area (m²) ______		area (m²/p)	______ (> 45)
	road access OK not OK	problem ______			
	water availability OK not OK	problem ______			
	drainage OK not OK	problem ______			
	building repair OK not OK	problem ______			
	electricity OK not OK	problem ______			
Issues	______				

Water	Lead Agency ________	Contact ________	Ph/Fax ________	
Indicators	site sources ________		open hours/d ____	
	# wells ____	# bladders/tanks ____	# taps or h pumps ____	
	condition of units ____	user fees Y N amount ____	p/tap or h pump ____	(< 250, 500)
	m to home ____ (< 500)	# users waiting ____	queue time (′) ____	(< 30)
	home sources ____	10-20 L sm neck containers Y N	overall L/p/d ____	(> 15)
	turbid Y N	color Y N	odor Y N	
	chlorination Y N	how ________	fecal coli/100 mL ____	(0)
Issues	________			
Sanitation	Lead Agency ________	Contact ________	Ph/Fax ________	
Indicators	# latrines ____	# full or blocked (0) ____	p/usable latrine ____	(< 20)
	latrine type and grouping ________		squat plate Y N	
	visible feces Y N	m from potable H_2O ____ (> 30)	m from dwelling ____	(< 50)
	handwash points Y N	type (tap, bucket) ________	soap gm/p/mo ____	(> 250)
	cleaning supplies Y N	maintenance teams Y N	printed health messages Y N	
	wash bucket Y N	p/wash basin ____ (< 100)	showers Y N	
	refuse drums Y N	families/drum ____ (< 10)	waste pit - dwelling (m)	
	vermin/vectors Y N	type ________	eradication activities Y N	
Issues	________			

Food/Nutrition	Lead Agency ________	Contact ________	Ph/Fax ________
Indicators	current foods ________		kcals/p/d ______ (> 2,100)
	household stores Y N	recent changes Y N	food security Y N
	food income (5 sources)	crops Y N	livestock Y N
	labor exchange Y N	wild foods Y N	relief Y N
	cash income (5 sources)	crops Y N	livestock Y N
	labor Y N	borrowing Y N	selling other assets Y N
	food distribution Y N	type, quantity, frequency ________	
	markets with food Y N	communal kitchen Y N	family kitchen & fuel Y N
Issues	________		
Non-Food	Lead Agency ________	Contact ________	Ph/Fax ________
Indicators	mats/mattresses Y N	blankets Y N	kitchen sets Y N
	hygiene parcels Y N	warehoused supplies Y N	kinds ________
Issues	________		
Shelter	Lead Agency ________	Contact ________	Ph/Fax ________
Indicators	# tents ______	# buildings ______	building materials ________
	sheeting Y N	bednets used Y N	shelter m^2/p ______ (> 3.5)
Issues	________		
Health	Lead Agency ________	Contact ________	Ph/Fax ________
Indicators	clinic on site Y N	time/distance from camp ______	days/hours open ________
	structure ok Y N	# doctors ______ # nurses ______	# CHWs ______ # TBAs ______
	running water Y N	toilet/latrine Y N	electricity Y N

	exam rooms ______	ORS corner Y N	overnight stay Y N
	dispensary Y N	drug shortages Y N	IV fluid Y N
	sharps container Y N	med waste disposal ______	handwashing Y N
	comms Y N	referral transport Y N	treatment fees Y N
	standard case defs Y N	treatment protocols Y N	stats reporting Y N
	case definition simple diarrhea ______		
	treatment simple pedes diarrhea ______		ORS prep demonstrated Y N
	patients understand mechanism of diarrhea transmission Y N		
	total visits/wk ______	active case finding Y N	% total pop/d ______ (< 1)
	total deaths/wk ______	active death finding Y N	deaths/10k p/d ______ (< 1)
	total referrals/wk ______	referral destination ______	diseases referred ______
Total # cases (past wk)	simple diarrhea ______	dysentery ______	visually confirmed Y N
	ARI ______	how diagnosed ______	(respiratory rate)
	measles ______	cold chain present Y N	date of last campaign ______
	malaria ______	how diagnosed ______	falciparum Y N
	malnutrition ______	type ______	nutrition program Y N
	trauma ______	type ______	
	psych ______	fear in population Y N	reason ______
	disease outbreaks Y N	type & date ______	epidemic control plan Y N
	provider stated needs ______		

Issues ______

Community Priorities	**Assessor Priorities**
1. ______	1. ______
2. ______	2. ______
3. ______	3. ______

Document 2.4
FEEDING CENTER ASSESSMENT

Date ______		Assessor ______	
Site Name ______		Informant #1 ______	
Location—GPS/landmark ______		Informant #2 ______	
Population	registration Y N	total pop ______	# households ______
	U1 ______ (5%)	women (15-44) ______ (20%)	arrivals/wk ______
	U5 ______ (20%)	men (15-44) ______ (10%)	departures/wk ______
	5-14 ______ (35%)	45+ ______ (15%)	typical livelihood ______
	vulnerable groups ______		
Security	Officer in Charge ______	Camp Leader ______	
Indicators	incidents at site Y N type (murder, rape, assault) ______		
Issues	______		
Site Mgmt	Lead Agency ______	Contact ______	Ph/Fax ______
Indicators	original site use ______	area (m^2) ______	area (m^2/p) ______ (> 45)
	road access OK not OK	problem ______	
	water availability OK not OK	problem ______	
	drainage OK not OK	problem ______	
	building repair OK not OK	problem ______	
	electricity OK not OK	problem ______	
Issues	______		

Water	Lead Agency ______	Contact ______	Ph/Fax ______
Indicators	site sources ______		open hours/d ______
	# wells ______	# bladders/tanks ______	# taps or h pumps ______
	condition of units ______	user fees Y N amount ______	p/tap or h pump ______ (< 250, 500)
	m to home ______ (< 500)	# users waiting ______	queue time (′) ______ (< 30)
	home sources ______	10-20 L sm neck containers Y N	overall L/p/d ______ (> 30)
	turbid Y N	color Y N	odor Y N
	chlorination Y N	how ______	fecal coli/100 mL ______ (0)
Issues	______		

Sanitation	Lead Agency ______	Contact ______	Ph/Fax ______
Indicators	# latrines ______	# full or blocked ______ (0)	p/usable latrine ______ (< 20)
	latrine type and grouping ______		squat plate Y N
	visible feces Y N	m from potable H_2O ______ (> 30)	m from dwelling ______ (< 50)
	handwash points Y N	type (tap, bucket) ______	soap gm/p/mo ______ (> 250)
	cleaning supplies Y N	maintenance teams Y N	printed health messages Y N
	wash bucket Y N	p/wash basin ______ (< 100)	showers Y N
	refuse drums Y N	families/drum ______ (< 10)	waste pit - dwelling (m) ______ (< 100)
	vermin/vectors Y N	type ______	eradication activities Y N
Issues	______		

Nutrition Lead Agency ____ Contact ____ Ph/Fax ____

Indicators
date opened ____ hours open ____ staffing ____
admission criteria ____
current phase 1 census U5 ____ O5 ____ Total ____
current transition census U5 ____ O5 ____ Total ____
current phase 2 census U5 ____ O5 ____ Total ____
admissions last week U5 ____ O5 ____ Total ____
cumulative admissions U5 ____ O5 ____ Total ____
trend analysis ____
coverage ____ (rural > 50%, urban > 70%, camp > 90%) active case finding Y N
estimated unmet needs ____
medical protocol Y N reference ____
hypoglycemia, hypothermia—D10 or F75
ABC (dehydration, sepsis)—ReSoMal or RL + D5 or ORS
GI (feeds)—F75 (initial), F100 +/- solid food (recovery)
ID (3)—antibiotics (TMP/SMZ), antihelminths (mebendazole), +/- antimalarials
adjuncts—vitamins A-D, minerals, measles vaccine, Fe (only in rehab phase)
underlying illnesses malaria Y N % ____ TB/HIV Y N % ____
referrals out Y N number last week ____ destination ____
discharge criteria ____
disposition ____
cure rate ____ (> 75%) death rate ____ (< 10%) default rate ____ (< 15%)
provider stated needs ____

Issues ____

Health Lead Agency ____ Contact ____ Ph/Fax ____

Indicators
clinic on site Y N time/distance from camp ____ days/hours open ____
structure ok Y N # doctors ____ # nurses ____ # CHWs ____ # TBAs ____
running water Y N toilet/latrine Y N electricity Y N

	exam rooms ______	ORS corner Y N	overnight stay Y N
	dispensary Y N	drug shortages Y N	IV fluid Y N
	sharps container Y N	med waste disposal ______________	handwashing Y N
	comms Y N	referral transport Y N	treatment fees Y N
	standard case defs Y N	treatment protocols Y N	stats reporting Y N
	case definition simple diarrhea ______________________________		
	treatment simple pedes diarrhea ______________________________		ORS prep demonstrated Y N
	patients understand mechanism of diarrhea transmission Y N		
	total visits/wk ______	active case finding Y N	% total pop/d ______ (< 1)
	total deaths/wk ______	active death finding Y N	deaths/10k p/d ______ (< 1)
	total referrals/wk ______	referral destination ______________	diseases referred ______________
Total # cases (past wk)	simple diarrhea ______	dysentery ______	visually confirmed Y N
	ARI ______	how diagnosed ______________	(respiratory rate)
	measles ______	cold chain present Y N	date of last campaign ______________
	malaria ______	how diagnosed ______________	falciparum Y N
	malnutrition ______	type ______________	nutrition program Y N
	trauma ______	type ______________	
	psych ______	fear in population Y N	reason ______________
	disease outbreaks Y N	type & date ______________	epidemic control plan Y N
	provider stated needs ______________________________		

Issues ____

Community Priorities

1. ______________________________
2. ______________________________
3. ______________________________

Assessor Priorities

1. ______________________________
2. ______________________________
3. ______________________________

Document 2.5a
ESTIMATES OF DISASTER-AFFECTED POPULATION

Source: Ministry of ______________, Capital City

Date ______

Location	Population per Census of Year	Humanitarian Assistance		Vulnerable Populations			Missing or unaccounted	Injured	Dead
		In Need	Targeted	Undisplaced	IDPs	Returnees			
Total									

Document 2.5b
ESTIMATES OF DISASTER-AFFECTED VULNERABLE GROUPS

Source: Ministry of ________________________ , Capital City

Date __________

Vulnerable Groups	Total Number	Humanitarian Assistance		Vulnerable Populations			Missing or unaccounted	Injured	Dead
		In Need	Targeted	Undisplaced	IDPs	Returnees			
U5									
malnourished									
orphaned									
abandoned									
pregnant									
lactating									
disabled									
elderly									
Total									

Document 2.5c
DAMAGE ESTIMATES

Source: Ministry of ______________________ , Capital City

Location ___________ Date ___________

Structure	Preexisting	Damaged		Functional	
		Destroyed # (%)	Hi/Med/Low # (%)	Partially # (%)	Fully # (%)
Residential					
Commercial					
Industrial					
Hazardous Materials					
Subtotal or %					
Public Bldgs					
Govt Admin					
Hospitals					
Health Centers					
Schools					
Community Shelters					
Police Stations					
Fire Stations					
Subtotal or %					
Lifelines				% Population with access	
				Partial	Full
Telecomms Landlines Mobiles					
Transport Road Rail Air					
Power supply					
Water supply					
Septic system					

Document 2.6a
SECTORAL GAP IDENTIFICATION

Function	Site 1	Site 2	Site 3	Site 4
Site Management				
Protection / Registration				
Security				
Logistics and Transport				
Water				
Sanitation				
Food Aid				
Non-Food Aid				
Shelter				
Health				
Education and Training				
Early Recovery				
Other				

Document 2.6b
HEALTH SECTOR GAP IDENTIFICATION

Function	Site 1	Site 2	Site 3	Site 4
Sector Management				
Immunization				
Clinical Health Services Health Center/Post				
Clinical Health Services Mobile clinics				
Clinical Health Services Hospital				
Clinical Pathology Laboratory support				
Special Services Reproductive health				
Special Services Maternal-child health				
Special Services Mental health				
Special Services HIV/AIDS				

Special Services **Nutrition**				
Epidemic Preparedness				
Communicable Disease Control				
Community Health Education				
Epidemiological Surveillance				
Medical Logistics				
Other				
Other				

3 Field Recommendations

Contents

Overview

This section provides guidance on recommendations for post-disaster field intervention. Recommendations fall prey to many feasibility traps—technical, administrative, political, economic, and developmental among them. Moreover, temporary solutions tend to become permanent. Hence, disaster decision-making requires impulse control and considered thought before action. Health determinants extend beyond the health sector per se—particularly in security and environmental health. Hence, these are critical loci of post-disaster interventions. "Unmet needs" is a core concept that devolves from quantifying needs offset by coping strategy and ongoing assistance. Public health interventions remain among the most cost-effective in the post-disaster health sector. By contrast, clinical interventions commonly seen after disasters are often not cost-effective—particularly when piggybacked on platforms such as disaster medical assistance teams, foreign field hospitals, or hospital ships.

Beneficiary unmet needs, agency mandate, political pressures, and resource availability may all influence the exact priority of recommendations submitted. Nonetheless, multi-party needs assessments should drive field responses, and recommendations should reflect beneficiary unmet needs. State them candidly and clearly. Above the medical coordinator in the organization's chain of command, no one else will have more insight or legitimacy in characterizing those needs.

D. A. Bradt, C. M. Drummond, *Pocket Field Guide for Disaster Health Professionals*,
https://doi.org/10.1007/978-3-030-04801-3_3

This section focuses on information priorities and health intervention priorities.

- Information priorities
  - Safety and security
  - Intervenors
  - Rapid epidemiological assessment and GIS information
  - Environmental health subsector information
  - Health subsector information

- Intervention priorities
  - Public health services
  - Health facilities and clinical services
  - Human resources
  - Essential medical products and technologies
  - Health information systems
  - Health financing
  - Health leadership and governance

Document 3.1
RAPID EPIDEMIOLOGICAL ASSESSMENT RECOMMENDATIONS

Date

XIII. RECOMMENDATIONS (copy to Exec Summary)

A. Information Priorities

1. Security information (protection issues)
2. Safety information (hazard issues)
3. Intervenor information (4Ws)
4. REA information (health sector issues)
5. GIS data (location issues)
6. WASH subsector analysis
   a. water (tanker) distribution system
   b. water quality testing findings
   c. HH water storage findings
7. Food security subsector analysis
   a. VAM (WFP), IPC, or FEWS NET analysis
   b. pipeline analysis
   c. market analysis
   d. transfer modality analysis
8. Health subsector surveys & surveillance
   a. epidemiological surveillance (EWARS, q 1 wk)
   b. health facilities and provider survey (HeRAMS, q 3 mo)
   c. nutritional survey (U5 WHZ, q 6 mo)
   d. immunization survey (U5 EPI, annual)
   e. communicable disease control survey (disease-specific)
   f. vector survey (presence, speciation, pathogen detection, eradication plan)
   g. medical logistics survey

B. Health Intervention Priorities (activities, not objectives)

Priority sectors: unmet needs per gap analysis with attention to:
List 1: initial assessment, measles immunization, water and sanitation, food and nutrition, shelter and site planning, health care, control of communicable diseases and epidemics, public health surveillance, human resources and training, coordination (MSF [1])
List 2: adequate shelter, sufficient safe food, sufficient sate water, sanitation facilities, environmental sanitation and waste disposal, mass vaccination, primary health care and referral care, disease surveillance and outbreak control, vector control, and health education and social mobilization (HPN [2])

1. Public health services
   a. disease prevention
      (1) primary prevention
         (a) measles immunization (6 mo – 12 yr (MSF); 6 mo - 5 yr (CDC); coverage >90%)
            (i) vaccine stocks
            (ii) cold chain
         (b) vitamin A distribution
         (c) restart EPI
      (2) communicable disease control (CDs of epidemic potential)
         (a) diarrhea
         (b) ARI
         (c) malaria
         (d) HIV
         (e) TB
         (f) other
   b. epidemiological surveillance (key data on health status, nutritional status, or health program activity)
      (1) data sources
         (a) provider-based alert system (24 h notice for notifiable conditions)
         (b) camp-based weekly system (esp from larger camps >2,500 p)
         (c) facility-based weekly system (from IPDs and OPDs)
         (d) lab-based weekly system (isolation and identification)
         (e) other relevant epi data—rumor and outbreaks
      (2) surveillance system components
         (a) clinical case definitions
         (b) camp logbooks
         (c) weekly surveillance report forms
         (d) reporting process—description and diagram
   c. epidemic preparedness and response
      (1) plan of action and coordinating committee
         (a) public health incident command system (PHICS)
         (b) cholera command and control center (C4)
      (2) clinical case definitions
      (3) case mgmt guidelines for communicable diseases with epidemic potential
      (4) outbreak mgmt protocol
         (a) surveillance definitions
         (b) alert thresholds
         (c) rapid response teams to investigate case reports
         (d) epidemic investigation kits to use
         (e) specimens to collect
         (f) labs to verify diagnosis (including sample sharing for confirmatory testing)

(g) patients to identify, isolate, and treat (inpatient and outpatient settings)
(i) isolation areas to organize
(ii) treatments to plan
(h) contacts to trace and ? quarantine
(i) hotlines to use for notifiable diseases and rumor investigation
(5) primary and secondary prevention
(a) infection control protocols
(b) commodities
(i) vaccines (eg measles, meningitis)
(ii) drugs (eg prophylactic meds)
(iii) chemicals (eg soap, calcium hypochlorite)
(iv) supplies (eg chlorimetric and colimetric monitors)
(v) equipment (eg PPE)
(6) resource prepositioning (stockpiles, supply chain)
(7) information mgmt and crisis communication (media strategy)
(a) health authorities, WHO
(b) political authorities
(c) community leaders and public
(i) social mobilization
(ii) hygiene promotion and health education
(iii) behavioral change communication (BCC)
(8) contingency planning for epidemic consequences
(a) provision of essential services (lifelines)
(b) corpse mgmt
d. health promotion (relevant to disaster response)
(1) targeted diseases
(a) acute epidemic diseases
(b) chronic diseases—HTN, DM, HIV/TB, asthma
(2) health promotion activities
(a) community health education
(b) provider education
e. health protection (relevant to disaster response)
(1) air quality (eg wildfires, volcanic eruptions)
(2) injury control
(3) occupational health and safety
(4) hazardous materials (eg chemical releases)
(5) disaster risk reduction (eg safe hospitals)
2. Health facilities and clinical services
a. vulnerable groups (IDPs/refugees on the move > IDPs/refugees in camps > IDPs/refugees in host communities > host country nationals staying put)
b. access to care
c. clinical epidemiology

- (1) ID
  - (a) diarrhea
  - (b) ARI
  - (c) malaria
  - (d) measles
  - (e) epidemic diseases
- (2) malnutrition
- (3) trauma
- (4) mental illness
- (5) chronic diseases

d. delivery of health services

- (1) stabilize and evacuate critical patients
- (2) restore workforce (staff need to care for their own families)
  - (a) redistribute host country staff
  - (b) use task shifting
  - (c) encourage incentives (recognition, benefits, payments)
  - (d) provide health situation updates for providers
- (3) initiate/restore levels of care and referral system
  - (a) home visiting by CHWs referring to health clinic
    - (i) active case finding
    - (ii) ORS and soap distribution
    - (iii) referral for immunization and key clinical symptoms
    - (iv) health education
    - (v) defaulter follow-up
  - (b) mobile clinics referring to fixed clinic
  - (c) fixed clinics referring to health center
  - (d) health centers referring to district hospital
  - (e) emergency medical teams & foreign field hospitals linked to referral system
- (4) initiate/restore primary, preventive, and basic services
  - (a) comprehensive primary health care (focusing on community-based interventions, health education, and standardized case management)
    - (i) SPHC as needed in severe resource-limited settings
  - (b) child health services
    - (i) EPI
    - (ii) IMCI
    - (iii) protection
  - (c) reproductive health services
    - (i) identify RH lead agency
    - (ii) prevent and manage consequences of SGBV (IASC Guidelines)
      - (a) acute trauma care
      - (b) emergency contraception (post rape)
      - (c) post-exposure prophylaxis
      - (d) psyc follow-up

(iii) reduce HIV transmission (IASC Guidelines)
(a) abstain, be faithful, use condoms (ABCs)
(b) standard precautions
(c) treatment of STIs
(d) PMTCT
(iv) safe motherhood—basic & comprehensive emergency obstetric care (IMPAC programs)
(a) antenatal care
(b) professional midwifery (midwifery kits)
(c) clean delivery (clean delivery kits)
(d) essential newborn care (warming and exclusive breast feeding)
(e) referral options
(v) family planning—plan for comprehensive RH services in PHC
(a) general contraception
(d) trauma services
(i) field stabilization
(ii) evacuation
(iii) initial facility care including damage control surgery
(iv) inter-hospital referral & definitive care
(v) rehabilitation
(vi) cost recovery
(e) mental health services (IASC Guidelines & Action Sheets)
(i) coordination
(ii) assessment, monitoring, & evaluation
(iii) protection & human rights standards
(iv) human resources
(v) community support
(vi) health services
(vii) education
(viii) dissemination
(f) chronic diseases (prioritize resource requirements beyond EHKs)
(5) reinforce standardized case management
(a) clinical case definitions
(b) treatment protocols (ORS + Zn, ABX, ACT, IPT, and ITN will save 75% of U5 deaths)
(c) other clinical protocols
(i) standard precautions
(ii) injection safety
(iii) medical waste mgmt
(d) essential (standard) drugs and rational drug use
(i) EHKs, National Pharmaceutical Stockpile push packs
(ii) specialty kits (including chronic disease kit)
(e) referral guidelines
(f) secondary prevention

   (6) reinforce infection control
      (a) dedicated staff
      (b) hand washing facilities
      (c) stocks of essential supplies (soap, gloves, masks, gowns)
      (d) infection control protocols (medical waste mgmt, safe transfusion)

3. Human resources
   a. areas and services in need
   b. sources of staff
   c. salaries/incentives for staff
   d. security for staff
4. Essential medical products and technologies (medical logistics)
   a. national formulary
   b. warehouse security
   c. storage of commodities completely in warehouse
   d. arrangements of pallets and shelves
   e. inventory system with stock cards—especially for drugs (SUMA)
   f. documentation of inflows and outflows
   g. central reporting
   h. supervision of peripheral facilities
   i. monitoring of aid distributions
5. Health information systems
   a. Vital statistics
   b. clinical
   c. laboratory
   d. epidemiological
   e. financial
6. Health financing
   a. subsidies
   b. costs, charges, and waivers
   c. provider incentives
7. Health leadership and governance
   a. key leaders
   b. technical support to coordination process

C. Other Sectoral Intervention Priorities

1. Security
   a. strategy
      (1) locate refugees/IDPs >20 km from borders and conflict areas
      (2) declare humanitarian corridors, pauses, and cease-fires
      (3) separate military from civilians (cantonment), and militias from non-combatants

   (4) disarm combatants (especially near refugees/IDPs)
   (5) demobilize military, disband militias (especially near refugees/IDPs)
   (6) repatriate, reintegrate former combatants in society of origin
   (7) arrest and prosecute perpetrators of violence
 b. military/police operations as needed
   (1) duty posts
   (2) checkpoints
   (3) patrols
   (4) vehicle escorts
   (5) camp management and civilian protection
   (6) safe havens
   (7) search and seizure of weapons
   (8) non-combatant evacuation
   (9) civil-military cooperation
     (a) central coordination
     (b) agreement on responsibilities and objectives
     (c) common territories of responsibility
     (d) compatible communications
     (e) collocation
     (f) liaison
     (g) inter-agency meetings
     (h) routine contacts between desk officers
     (i) civil-military operations centers
     (j) joint reconnaissance and assessments

2. Protection (who, where, from what)
 a. actors
   (1) civilian lead protection agency (UNHCR, OHCHR, OCHA)
     (a) monitor protection violations
     (b) document protection violations—incident lists, spot maps, and trend analysis
     (c) report events of concern to local authorities
     (d) review with host government
     (e) ensure follow-up
   (2) intervenor credentialing
   (3) refugees/IDPs
     (a) self-organization
     (b) go and see visits (respected refugee/IDP leaders visit country/area of origin)
     (c) come and talk visits (respected leaders from country/area of origin visit refugees/IDPs)
 b. protective programming
   (1) maintain access to refugees/IDPs (protection by presence)
   (2) register refugees/IDPs

(3) reunify families and undertake child tracing
(4) ensure refugees/IDPs participate in program decisions
(5) deploy dedicated protection officers
(6) identify the most vulnerable
(7) prevent SEA
(8) establish community watch (no relocations without consent)
(9) establish safety audits (q 3 mo)
(10) establish anonymous reporting
(11) establish a complaint and referral mechanism
(12) provide services and spaces for the most vulnerable without stigmatization
(a) child protection—child-friendly spaces
(b) SGBV—women's centers
(c) psychosocial services
(d) mental health services

c. health diplomacy (Health as a Bridge for Peace)
(a) humanitarian pauses
(b) humanitarian corridors
(c) medevac
(d) safe spaces, conflict exclusion zones
(i) immunization days
(ii) food distributions
(iii) NFI distributions
(iv) verification visits

3. Safety (for all parties to relief operation)
a. evacuation of civilians
b. personal protective equipment (PPE)
c. hazard-specific mitigation plans (see also C6)
4. Search and rescue (if ongoing)
5. Logistics (esp for relief agencies)
a. telecommunications plan
b. transportation, fuel
6. Environment
a. site-specific mitigation plans (see also C3)
b. site stabilization, drainage (with understanding of local conditions during seasonal weather changes)
7. Environmental health
a. water supply
(1) sources—near the people if possible; if not, bring it to the people rather than people to it. Aquifer > surface water.
(a) if aquifer—deep > shallow
(b) if surface—flowing > still
(2) access—monitor it vs patrol it vs guard it
(3) quantity (5 L/p/d initially → 15–20 L/p/d after 60 d)
(a) bucket distribution with hand chlorination
(b) jerry cans (20 L) with hand chlorination

- (c) tanker trucks (8,000 L) with chlorinated water
- (d) water bladders (3,000–10,000 L) with chlorinated water (500 p/d served by 10 MT bladder; 10 k p need 200 k L/d from 10×10 MT bladders filled 2×/d)
- (e) wells → handpumps (serve 500 p/d, require bucket chlorination) → submersible pumps (serve 5k p/d, enable batch chlorination)
- (f) boreholes with pumps > surface water treatment units
- (g) piped systems

(4) quality (0 coliforms/dL)

- (a) source protection (esp wells)
  - (i) separate surface water and defecation areas
  - (ii) fence to keep out animals
  - (iii) wall to keep out children
  - (iv) cover to keep out adults
  - (v) container which doesn't touch ground
  - (vi) channel for spill run-off
- (b) storage system protection
  - (i) cover on jars and jerry cans
  - (ii) personal hygiene
- (c) water purification (0.05 mg/dL free Cl, < 5 NTU)
  - (i) physical (boiling, filters—ceramic, sand, compressed clay + rice husk)
  - (ii) chemical (chlorination, alum flocculation; tankers vs on-site storage cisterns vs hand chlorination of household jerry cans and buckets)
  - (iii) radiological UV (SODIS)
  - (iv) combination (portable water purification units with filtration, flocculation, and chlorination—15,000 L/h)
  - (v) reverse osmosis

b. sanitation

priority populations

- new & existing IDP/refugee camps >
- host communities with IDPs/refugees where existing facilities are overtaxed >
- rural communities with IDP returns where rehab/reconstruction is needed and security is permissive

WASH presence distributed thru priority populations above plus health, nutrition, and women's centers

WASH programming comprehensively addressed at given site to include waste disposal (excreta, household, and solid waste), hand hygiene and bathing, hygiene kit distribution, and hygiene promotion integrating health and nutrition messages

(1) excreta disposal
  (a) facilities construction (50–100 p/latrine initially → 20 p/latrine after 60 d, < 50 m from housing, > 30 m from H_2O)
    (i) defecation fields (days)
    (ii) trench latrines (weeks)
    (iii) public pit latrines (weeks) (1 M p need 20 k latrines on 20 k m^2 space)
    (iv) family pit/raised latrines (depends on water table) (months)
    (v) pour flush (siphon) toilets (months)
    (vi) septic system (year)
  (b) hand hygiene
    (i) water points and soap (250 g bathing soap/p/mo, 200 g laundry soap/p/mo)
  (c) hygiene promotion
  (d) operations and maintenance
    (i) maintenance teams
    (ii) cleaning supplies
(2) garbage disposal
  (a) collection and removal
  (b) burial
(3) solid waste disposal
  (a) incineration
  (b) burial
(4) medical waste disposal
  (a) incineration
  (b) burial
(5) corpse management
  (a) disaster victim identification
  (b) disposal
    (i) cremation
    (ii) burial
(6) dead animal management
  (a) incineration
  (b) burial

c. food and nutrition
(1) beneficiary population (IPC 3+, GAM > 5%)
(2) assistance target (% of above)
(3) assistance ration (% of MDR; 50% is common for WFP)
(4) transfer modality
  (a) food (general food distribution)
  (b) food for assets (formerly food for work)
  (c) cash
  (d) voucher

(5) general food distribution
  (a) commodity basket standardization (based on family size and HIV status)
  (b) mechanism (0.5 kg/p/d, 15 kg/p/mo, 1 MT/1000 p/2 d, 15 MT/1000 p/mo, 450 MT/10,000 p/3 mo, 30,000 MT (prepo depot size)/2 M p/mo)
  NB plan depends on population distribution, disaster damage, security situation, and food distribution sites
    (i) humanitarian daily ration airdrops (Phase 1)
    (ii) bulk foods by helicopter (Phase 2)
    (iii) bulk foods by road (Phase 3)
(6) infant and young child feeding (IYCF)
(7) emergency school feeding (ESF)
(8) supplementary feeding program (> 350 kcal/p/d with RUSF—Plumpy'Sup®, high energy biscuits; priorities are U5 (6 mo – 5 yr) with GAM, pregnant (esp third trimester) or lactating women (esp 1st yr), medical referrals) (Sphere)
  (a) blanket SFP if GAM > 20% or > 10% if aggravating factors
  (b) targeted SFP if GAM > 10% or > 5% if aggravating factors
    coverage goals: > 50% in rural areas, > 70% in urban areas, > 90% in camp settings (Sphere)
  ∴ cure rate > 75%, CFR < 3%, defaulter rate < 15% (Sphere)
    aggravating factors = CMR > 1/10,000/day, basic ration inadequate, epidemic communicable disease, or severe cold
  NB no SFP if GAM < 5%
(9) therapeutic feeding program (where SAM > 2%, GAM > 10%; GAM > 15% is critical) (WHO)
  (a) TFC census should be <50 (WHO); if >50, add another site
  ∴ cure rate > 75%, CFR < 10%, defaulter rate < 15% (Sphere)
(10) market interventions to ensure food affordability
(11) inspection (regulatory control over farms, abattoirs, and restaurants)

d. shelter & settlements (emergency shelter → transitional shelter → permanent housing)
  (1) household shelter (in chronological order)
    (a) 1–3 mo: emergency shelter in place (salvaged materials, plastic sheeting, tarpaulins > tents (think outside the tent))

(b) 3–12 mo: hazard-resistant transitional shelter (rehabilitated shelter > prefabricated shelter b/c $300 to buy, $300 to ship)
(c) 12 mo +: permanent housing built back better (cement floor with corrugated sheet metal sides & roofing)

(2) settlement options
   (a) safe (home) site, same structures repaired
   (b) safe (home) plot, emergency or transitional shelter
   (c) host family
   (d) resettlement in safe proximity to destroyed home
   (e) resettlement in planned site (community/civic centers, schools, churches) for those without options a - d
   (f) resettlement in camps (always last choice)
(3) shelter package (if relief/rehab distribution is needed)
   (a) shelter repair kit, vouchers, or cash
   (b) non-food items
   (c) food basket
   (d) assisted utilities
   (e) debris removal
   (f) tents (always last choice)
(4) settlement development (if reconstruction solution can be staged)
   (a) wat/san
   (b) transportation hubs, communication links
   (c) homes, shop-homes
      (i) 1 family = 5 people
      (ii) 16 families = 80 people = 1 community
      (iii) 16 communities = 1250 people = 1 block/village
      (iv) 4 blocks = 5000 people = 1 sector
      (v) 4 sectors = 20,000 people = 1 camp
   (d) shops, stalls, and kiosks
   (e) health facilities
   (f) other civil buildings
(5) plan for permanent shelter using DRR best practices
   (a) hazard-resistant design
   (b) training in hazard-resistant construction
   (c) public information campaigns on building back better

e. emergency relief supplies (non food items)
   (1) plastic sheeting
   (2) blankets
   (3) jerry cans
   (4) cooking utensils
   (5) hygiene kits
   (6) mats

f. vector control/reservoir control
   (1) mosquitoes
      (a) insecticide treated nets
      (b) indoor residual spraying at beginning of transmission season (more effective in Asia than Africa; not appropriate for dengue)
      (c) drainage/elimination of breeding sites
      (d) larvicide in standing water
      NB aerial spraying, outdoor spraying (fogging) are not really useful
   (2) rodents
      (a) food storage
      (b) garbage disposal

8. Additional common concerns
   a. public utility restoration
      (1) power supply
      (2) water supply
      (3) excreta disposal/septic systems
   b. resource prepositioning
      (1) resource type
      (2) feasibility of sourcing it
      (3) feasibility of transporting, storing, and protecting it
   c. relocation (if security, environment, or environmental health incompatible with local human habitation)
      (1) impact study (esp on land use and socio-economic issues in receiving areas)
      (2) formal plan with contingency plan to scale back in event of problems
      (3) government led coordination body to establish minimum standards
      (4) donors and implementing partners involved in planning and agreed on standards
      (5) informed consent
      (6) family unification
      (7) reciprocal visits prior to relocation (reps to sending and receiving areas) with information campaign to avert rumor
      (8) basic infrastructure in place prior to relocation (feeder roads, water points, health clinics, schools)
      (9) safe transport to resettlement sites with transit centers en route
      (10) safety net for settlers
         (a) cash or food rations until next harvest (donor will not want this)
         (b) land enabling agricultural self-sufficiency
         (c) draft animals, seeds, and tools on grant basis
         (d) social services for settlers and local communities
      (11) external monitoring

D. Coordination Priorities

1. Cluster/sector dedicated full-time coordinator
2. NGO co-lead
3. Cluster SAGs and TWiGs
4. Inter-cluster working group
5. Cluster work products
6. Rapid response mechanism to assess and deliver
7. L3 status for individual UN lead agencies
8. Stand-by partnerships to mobilize staff as needed
9. Scale up for IASC system as a whole
10. Peer review
    a. Operational Peer Review (OPR) (90 d) and L3 transitions
    b. Emergency Directors' Group site visits
    c. Inter-agency Humanitarian Evaluation (12 m)

E. Program Implementation

1. Reallocation of existing local & national resources
2. Revision/refinement of present (medical) practices
    a. use of essential drugs
    b. use of standardized case management
    c. elimination of dated practices
3. Financial assistance (critical funding)
4. Technical assistance (critical skills)
    a. complement donated goods
    b. support appropriate technology
    c. develop information systems
5. Material assistance (critical goods)
    a. essential drugs and vaccines
    b. consumable supplies
    c. other stated needs of health authorities
6. Provision of direct services (substitution)
7. Integration of programming
8. Coordination of external assistance
    NB cooperation = shared goals; coordination = shared tasks; collaboration = shared resources
    a. identification and registration of actors
    b. actor/area/activity (who/what/where) matrix
    c. gap analysis and priority setting
    d. establishment of rapid response mechanism
    e. gap filling via complementary inputs linking iNGOs & local NGOs to local health authorities
        (1) technical—staff mobilization
        (2) material—resource prepositioning and supply chain linkages
        (3) financial—external resource mobilization
    f. identification of deliverables and timetables

g. consolidated reporting and dissemination
   (1) group terms of reference
   (2) meeting minutes
   (3) epidemiology updates
   (4) health sitreps
   (5) component analysis
   (6) field documentation (toolkit) for new arrivals
9. Capacity building of host authorities
10. Civil society partnership and support
    a. organization of community leaders
    b. encourage gender mainstreaming
    c. encourage privatization
    d. discourage entitlements
11. Advocacy
12. Transition to early recovery
13. Monitoring and evaluation
    a. remote management system if needed
    b. risk management system to prevent and detect waste, fraud, and abuse

References

1. Médecins Sans Frontières. (1997). *Refugee health—An approach to emergency situations*. Hong Kong: Macmillan Education.
2. Checchi, F., Gayer, M., Grais, R. F., & Mills, E. J. (2007). Public health in crisis-affected populations—A practical guide for decision-makers. *Humanitarian Practice Network, Network Paper No 61, December 2007*. London: Overseas Development Institute.

Document 3.2 RECOMMENDATIONS SUMMARY WORKSHEET

A. Information Priorities

B. Health Intervention Priorities

1. Public health services
2. Health facilities and clinical services
3. Human resources
4. Essential medical products and technologies
5. Health information systems
6. Health financing
7. Health leadership and governance

C. Other Sectoral Intervention Priorities

1. Security
2. Protection
3. Safety
4. Search and rescue
5. Logistics
6. Environment
7. Environmental health

D. Coordination Priorities

4 Field Reporting

Contents

Overview

This section provides guidance on field reporting. The reporting burden can be eased by data gathering templates whose structure facilitates comprehensive and concise reporting afterward. While reporting is often viewed as a compliance burden, it should be viewed as a leadership opportunity to analyze field conditions and mobilize resources for response. What templates cannot provide is analytic insight. The greatest weakness in health situation reporting is poor data analysis. Field grade insight with cost-effective recommendations are the hallmarks of competent medical coordinators.

This section focuses on 3 main reporting instruments.

- Rapid epidemiological assessment report
  REA report derives from REA (Sect. 2) and Recommendations (Sect. 3). It is generally supplemented by an executive summary at the beginning and document annexes at the end.
- Weekly health situation report
  Health sitrep is generally produced weekly in the acute disaster setting. It focuses on updates and new findings. Template details are not intended to be prescriptive, but rather probative in coherent ways. If no new details emerge that week, that that part of the report is summarized as "nothing new" or suppressed altogether.

D. A. Bradt, C. M. Drummond, *Pocket Field Guide for Disaster Health Professionals*,
https://doi.org/10.1007/978-3-030-04801-3_4

- Health sector status summary
  Status summary tabulates subsector lead agency, milestones and benchmarks, current status, and overall priority/unmet need. These summaries are a 3-fold opportunity:
  - the leadership opportunity to quickly demonstrate an ability to organize cross-cutting information relevant to numerous stakeholders in the disaster response;
  - the strategic opportunity to shape the optics of disaster relief by proper prioritization of relief issues;
  - the tactical opportunity to quickly orient new staff to the field.

Document 4.1
RAPID EPIDEMIOLOGICAL ASSESSMENT REPORT

Date

EXECUTIVE SUMMARY

A. **Introduction** (copied from REA I A-B)

B. **REA Principal Findings and Analysis** (copied from REA XII)

C. **Recommendations** (copied from REA XIII)

I. INTRODUCTION

A. **Hazard History Abridged**

B. **Current Disaster**

C. **Immediate Response of Host Government Authorities**

D. **Your Mission**

II. SOURCES AND METHODS

A. **Assessment Team Composition**

B. **Assessment Area and Dates**

C. **Information Sources and Assessment Methods**

D. **Logistics of Assessment Team**

E. **Constraints**

III. PRE-EXISTING INDICATORS (summarize Tool 3.T1)

IV. DISASTER IMPACT

A. **Area Affected** (focus on most affected)

B. **Population Affected** (focus on most affected; see Tool 3.T2a, 3.T2b)

C. **Damage Assessment** (focus on most affected area; see Tool 3.T2c)

D. **Secondary Disasters and Threats**

E. **Disaster Impact Summary**

V. CURRENT EPIDEMIOLOGICAL INDICATORS

A. **Epidemiology**

B. **Outbreaks and Epidemics**

C. **Epidemiological Summary**

VI. HEALTH SECTOR FUNCTIONAL STATUS

A. Public Health Services (focus on service disruptions, adequacy)

1. Data
2. Issues summary

B. Health Facilities and Clinical Services (focus on service disruptions, adequacy; see Tool 3.T2c)

1. Data
2. Issues summary

C. Human Resources (focus on catchment area of interest)

1. Data
2. Issues summary

D. Essential Medical Products and Technologies

1. Data
2. Issues summary

E. Health Information Systems

1. Data
2. Issues summary

F. Health Financing (disaster-specific)

1. Data
2. Issues summary

G. Health Leadership and Governance

1. Data
2. Issues summary

H. Health Sector Functional Status Summary

VII. OTHER SECTORS

A. Security

1. Data
2. Issues summary

B. Protection (who, where, from what)

1. Data
2. Issues summary

C. Safety (for all parties to relief operation)

1. Data
2. Issues summary

D. Search and Rescue (if ongoing)

1. Data
2. Issues summary

E. Logistics (esp for relief agencies)

1. Data
2. Issues summary

F. Environment

1. Data
2. Issues summary

G. Environmental Health

1. Data
2. Issues summary

VIII. RESPONSE OF DOMESTIC (HOST COUNTRY) AUTHORITIES

A. Disaster Management Mechanism

B. Emergency Protection Powers in Disasters

C. Advisories and Decrees

D. Issues Summary

IX. RESPONSE OF INTERNATIONAL COMMUNITY

A. Coordination of International Assistance

B. Intervenors

C. Multi-party Assessments

D. International Appeals

E. Issues Summary

X. RESPONSE OF REPORTING AGENCY

A. Assessment Activities Undertaken

B. Assistance Projects/Activities Undertaken

C. Coordination of External Assistance

D. Collaboration in Partnership Development

E. Support to Civil Society

F. Transition to Early Recovery

G. Issues Summary

XI. OPERATIONAL CONSTRAINTS

A. Security

B. Political/Administrative

C. Logistical

D. Technical

E. Economic

F. Developmental

XII. REA PRINCIPAL FINDINGS AND ANALYSIS (list major findings from section summaries; emphasize summaries bolded below as most relevant to health sector; use phrases, not sentences)

A. Disaster Impact Summary (see REA IV E)

B. Epidemiological Summary (see REA V C)

C. Health Sector Functional Status Summary (see REA VI H)

D. Security, Protection, and Safety (see REA VII A,B,C)

E. Search and Rescue (see REA VII D)

F. Logistics (see REA VII E)

G. Environment (see REA VII F)

H. Environmental Health (see REA VII G)

I. Stated Needs of Health Authorities (see REA VIII A 10)

J. Major Gaps (see REA IX E)

K. Operational Constraints (see REA XI)

L. Duration of Emergency Phase (see REA VIII C1)

M. Future Risk Factors (see REA IV D)

XIII. RECOMMENDATIONS

A. Information Priorities

B. Health Intervention Priorities

C. Other Sectoral Intervention Priorities

D. Coordination Priorities

E. Program Implementation

XIV. DOCUMENTATION ANNEXES

A. Terms of Reference

B. List of Team Members (name, role, deployment location, time period)

C. List of Contacts (name, title, location)

D. Itinerary and Chronology (meetings, site visits)

E. Records and Reports

F. Surveys and Surveillance

G. Testimonies

H. Photographs and Maps

I. Other Primary and Secondary Source Documents

J. Technical Notes

K. Glossary (may place at beginning of report after Executive Summary)

Document 4.2
WEEKLY HEALTH SITUATION REPORT

Date

I. **SITUATION ON ARRIVAL** (1st report only)

A. **Disaster Impact** (see REA IV)

II. **CURRENT HEALTH INDICATORS**

A. **Population Affected**

1. Census
2. Location
3. Population movements

B. **Disease Surveillance Reporting**

1. Data sources
   a. report forms per ...
   b. case definitions per ...
2. Collection interval

C. **Epidemiology** (structure per REA V A)

1. Mortality
   a. total deaths, excess mortality
   b. proportional mortality
      (1) cause-specific proportion of D_T (diarrhea, measles have each caused up to 40% of D_T in acute emergencies)
      (2) D_T/P_T % (if $D_T \geq 1\%$ of P_T)
   c. death rates & trends
      (1) crude (< 1/10,000/d; > 2 is critical)
      (2) age-specific eg 0–5 DR (< 2/10,000/d; > 4 is critical) (often 50% of D_T)
      (3) disease-specific (uncommonly used)
      (4) excess (crisis death rate – baseline death rate)
   d. case-fatality ratios
      (1) diarrhea (cholera 2–50%, dysentery 2–20%; target is CFR < 1%)
      (2) ARI (pneumonia 2–20%)
      (3) malaria
      (4) measles (2–30%)
      (5) malnutrition (associated with 50% of U5 deaths)
      (6) trauma (20% of civilian injured in acute military conflict)

2. Morbidity
   a. total cases
   b. proportional morbidity
      (1) acute disease (epi estimates underlying early versions of EHKs)
         (a) adult presentations (1 adult obtains ~4 consults/yr; 5000 adults obtain ~5000 consults/3 mo)
         % adults presenting with: GI 25%, ARI 20%, MS 15%, GU 15%, malaria 10%, trauma 5%, anemia 5%, ocular 5%
         (b) pedes (1 child obtains ~5 consults/yr; 5000 children obtain ~6500 consults/3 mo)
         % pedes presenting with: GI 30%, ARI 30%, worms 20%, malaria 15%, trauma 10%, anemia 10%, ocular 10%, otic 5%
      (2) chronic disease (20% of P_T)
   c. incidence rates & trends
      (1) presentation rate/d (1% baseline - 10% in CDs)
      (2) age-specific (high risk = U5, O50)
      (3) disease-specific
         (a) diarrhea (AR 50%/mo in U5 excluding below)
            (i) dysentery (AR 5–30% over 1–3 mo in P_T)
            (ii) cholera (AR 1–5% over 1–4 mo in P_T)
         (b) ARI (AR 50%/mo in U5 esp in cold weather)
         (c) malaria (AR 50%/mo in P_T non-immune; 2%/mo in P_T immune (WHO))holo-endemic—intense transmission year-round (Congo)
         (6–10 infections/child/yr; mortality highest in U5 & preg F)
         hyper-endemic—intense transmission seasonally (W. Afr) (4–6 infections/child/yr; mortality across all ages)
         hypo-endemic—low transmission year-round (Thai-Burma) (1 infection/person/yr; mortality across all ages)
         (d) measles (AR 10%/epidemic in U12 non-immunized; 10–75% of cases with complications depending on health status)
         (e) malnutrition
            (i) macro (PEM 10% with $Z < -2$, 1% with $Z < -3$)
            (ii) micro (vitamins A-D; Fe, I)
         (f) trauma
            (i) (para)military conflict
            (ii) rape
            (iii) domestic violence
            (iv) motor vehicle trauma

(g) mental health
   (i) adjustment disorders (debilitating grief reactions)
   (ii) psychiatric disease
   (iii) violence
   (iv) drug abuse

D. Outbreaks and Epidemics (structure per REA V B, or update since last report)

1. Recent or ongoing
   a. etiology
   b. date of first case(s)
   c. location
   d. number of cases or attack rate
   e. consequences or current status
2. Potential
   a. wide geographic relevance
      (1) measles
      (2) cholera (dehydrating diarrhea)
      (3) shigella (bloody diarrhea)
      (4) meningococcus (meningitis)
      (5) hepatitis A, E (acute jaundice syndrome)
      (6) influenza
   b. specific geographic relevance
      (1) malaria
      (2) viral hemorrhagic fevers (eg yellow fever, lassa fever, dengue HF)
      (3) typhoid (FUO)
      (4) leishmaniasis
      (5) polio
      (6) other (eg typhus, plague)
   c. specific age groups
      (1) polio (acute flaccid paralysis)
      (2) neonatal tetanus

E. Epidemiological Summary

III. HEALTH SECTOR FUNCTIONAL STATUS (structure per REA VI, or update since last report)

A. Public Health Services (focus on service disruptions, adequacy)

1. Disease prevention
   a. primary prevention
      (1) measles vaccination
      (2) EPI restart
      (3) other epidemic diseases

   b. communicable disease control programs
      (1) diarrhea
      (2) ARI
      (3) malaria
      (4) HIV
      (5) TB
      (6) other
2. Epidemiological surveillance system
   a. system objectives
   b. health events/indicator conditions and case definitions
   c. system components and flow chart of operations
   d. level of usefulness
   e. system attributes
   f. system resource requirements
3. Epidemic preparedness and response
   a. plan of action and coordinating committee
      (1) public health incident command system (PHICS)
      (2) cholera command and control center (C4)
   b. clinical case definitions
   c. case mgmt guidelines for communicable diseases with epidemic potential
   d. outbreak mgmt protocol
      (1) surveillance definitions
      (2) alert thresholds
      (3) rapid response teams to investigate case reports
      (4) epidemic investigation kits to use
      (5) specimens to collect
      (6) labs to verify diagnosis (including sample sharing for confirmatory testing)
      (7) patients to identify, isolate, and treat (inpatient and outpatient settings)
         (a) isolation areas to organize
         (b) treatments to plan
      (8) contacts to trace and ? quarantine
      (9) hotlines to use for notifiable diseases and rumor investigation
   e. primary and secondary prevention
      (1) infection control protocols
      (2) commodities
         (a) vaccines (eg measles, meningitis)
         (b) drugs (eg prophylactic meds)
         (c) chemicals (eg soap, Ca hypochlorite)
         (d) supplies (eg chlorimetric and colimetric monitors)
         (e) equipment (eg PPE)

(f) resource prepositioning (stockpiles, supply chain)
(g) information mgmt and crisis communication (media strategy)
    (1) health authorities, WHO
    (2) political authorities
    (3) community leaders and public
        (a) social mobilization
        (b) hygiene promotion and health education
        (c) behavioral change communication (BCC)
(h) contingency planning for epidemic consequences (ref DHHS flu pandemic plan)
    (1) provision of essential services (lifelines)
    (2) corpse mgmt

4. Health promotion (relevant to disaster response)
    a. targeted diseases
        (1) acute epidemic diseases
        (2) chronic diseases—HTN, DM, HIV/TB, asthma
    b. health promotion activities
        (1) community health education
        (2) provider education
5. Health protection (relevant to disaster response)
    a. air quality (eg wildfires, volcanic eruptions)
    b. injury control
    c. occupational health and safety
    d. hazardous materials (eg chemical releases)
    e. disaster risk reduction (eg safe hospitals)

B. Health Facilities and Clinical Services (focus on service disruptions, adequacy)

	Fixed Clinics	Health Centers	District Hospitals
1. Health facilities			
2. Clinical services			
3. Special services			
a. child health			
b. reproductive health			
c. trauma			
d. mental health			
e. chronic diseases			
4. Case management			
5. Infection control			

C. Human Resources

1. Additions and subtractions since last report

D. Essential Medical Products and Technologies (status, new issues)

E. Health Information Systems (status, new issues)

F. Health Financing (status, new issues)

G. Health Leadership and Governance (status, new issues)

IV. OTHER SECTORS (structure per REA VII, or update since last report)

A. Security

B. Protection (who, where, from what)

C. Safety (for all parties to relief operation)

D. Search and Rescue (if relevant to relief operation)

E. Logistics

F. Environment

G. Environmental Health

V. RESPONSE OF DOMESTIC AUTHORITIES

A. Key Decisions and Actions

B. Adequacy of Coordination

VI. RESPONSE OF INTERNATIONAL COMMUNITY

A. Updates from HC, HCT, ICCG

B. Status of Appeals

C. New Actors

VII. RESPONSE OF REPORTING AGENCY—PROGRAM IMPLEMENTATION

A. Brief Analysis of External Situation

B. Project-specific Outputs

1. Direct services to beneficiaries
2. Indirect services to beneficiaries
   a. Rapid epidemiological assessment
   b. Inter-agency medical coordination
   c. Standardized case management
   d. Environmental health
   e. Epidemic preparedness and response

f. Disease surveillance
g. Special surveys
h. Health policy and personnel planning
i. Immunization programs
j. Medical logistics
k. Hazard specific issues
3. Capacity building

C. Resource Management

1. Human resources
   a. team structure and function
   b. staff presence (quantify)
      (1) R&R schedules
      (2) incoming briefings
      (3) end-of-mission debriefings
   c. upcoming staff selection
      (1) internationals
      (2) local staff
   d. major gaps
2. Material resources
   a. major gaps
3. Financial resources
   a. major gaps
4. Donations
   a. Medical consumables
   b. IT
   c. Other in-kind

D. New Assessments

E. Operational Constraints

1. Security
2. Political/Administrative
3. Logistical (operational support)
   a. comms
   b. transport
   c. office set-up
   d. food and lodging
4. Technical
5. Economic
6. Developmental

F. VIP Visitors

G. Team Safety and Health

1. Safety & security plan
   a. SOPs
      (1) activities of daily living
      (2) warden system
      (3) vehicle safety
      (4) office safety
      (5) residential safety
2. Communications plan
3. Staff health emergency plan
   a. staff health records
   b. prophylaxis (eg malaria)
   c. field medical care
   d. medevac
4. Contingency plans
   a. fire
   b. individual adverse events (kidnapping, carjacking)
   c. security instability (eg insurgent attack)
   d. team evacuation plan

H. Meetings Held

I. Work Products Produced

J. Leadership Opportunities

K. Upcoming Deadlines and Explosive Issues

VIII. FUTURE PLANS/NEXT STEPS

A. Information Needs

B. Intervention Plans

C. Inputs Required

1. Staff (position, where, when, TOR)
2. Material
3. Financial

D. Follow-up

Document 4.3
HEALTH SECTOR STATUS SUMMARY

Site: ____________ **Date:** ____________

Components of Assistance	Milestones and Benchmarks	Status	Priority	Lead/Contact
Rapid Epidemiological Assessment and Monitoring				
Security	Humanitarian space accessible			
Communication	Radio handset provision			
Transport	Vehicles available, suitable for terrain			
Beneficiary identification and access	1. Site mapping			
	2. Registration			
Rapid epidemiological assessment	Template			
Assessment priorities	Population size, vulnerability, M & M			
Public Health and Clinical Services				
Immunization	1. Measles coverage rate			
	2. Vitamin A distribution			
Clinical services	Complete camp/site allocation			
PHC	Service delivery			
Mobile clinics	Service delivery			
Hospitals	Service delivery			

Standardized case management	1. Clinical case definitions			
	2. Treatment protocols			
	3. Essential drugs			
	4. Referral guidelines			
	5. Secondary prevention measures			
Special needs				
Reproductive health	Service delivery—MISP, SGBV			
Maternal-child health	Service delivery			
Mental health	Service delivery			
HIV/AIDS	Service delivery—VCT, PMTCT, SCM			
Trauma care	Service delivery—EMS to rehab			
Epidemic preparedness				
Comm. diseases of epidemic potential	Clinical case definitions			
	Case management guidelines			
Outbreak management protocol	1. Rapid response team to investigate			
	2. Specimen collection protocol to follow			
	3. Reference lab to identify			
	4. Patients to isolate			
	5. Contact tracing			

(continued)

Components of Assistance	Milestones and Benchmarks	Status	Priority	Lead/Contact
Communicable disease control				
EPI	National program			
Malaria	National program			
TB/HIV	National program			
Community Health Education	Culturally appropriate messages			
Quality improvement	Site monitoring visits			
Epidemiological Surveillance				
Data source identification	Reporting sites			
Data management	1. Routine epi data flow			
	2. Data collection and analysis			
	3. Reporting and dissemination			
Special surveys	Methodology			
Environmental Health Services				
Water supply	Minimum standards			
Food supply	Minimum standards			
Supplementary feeding	Minimum standards			
Sanitation	Minimum standards			
Shelter	Minimum standards			
Vector control	Service delivery			

Health Sector Coordination				
Inventory of organizations	Contact list			
Cluster/sectoral coordination meetings	Schedule			
Health system catchments	Defined			
Agency area-specific task designations	Operational mapping with PHA/DHA			
Health personnel/team credentialing	Defined process			
Drug importation/medical logistics	Defined process			
Provincial health authority capacity bldg	Self-sufficient health sector mgmt			
Contingency planning	Plan developed and disseminated			

Compiled: ____________________

Source: adapted from D Bradt, C Drummond in *Prehospital and Disaster Medicine* © 2003. Used with permission

5 Field Project and Staff Management

Contents

Overview

This section provides guidance on field project and staff management. Project planning is complicated. Before going to the field, it is helpful to be familiar with planning precursors such as context analysis, stakeholder analysis, SWOT analysis, and force field analysis. It is also helpful to be familiar with planning tools such as problem trees, objective trees, project maps, logframes, and workplans. Certain planning steps have particular boundary conditions or sensitivities for an organization. Director's input is especially important in establishing priorities, selecting a strategy, and developing a budget.

This section focuses on developing a project plan of action with its associated logframe. The use of a logframe may not improve the quality of services described in a proposal. However, it will improve funding prospects with a serious donor. Health personnel tend to focus on the service end of a project rather than the procurement end. They should pay attention to medical logistics. Amateurs discuss strategy, but professionals discuss logistics.

D. A. Bradt, C. M. Drummond, *Pocket Field Guide for Disaster Health Professionals*,
https://doi.org/10.1007/978-3-030-04801-3_5

Document 5.1
PROJECT PLANNING OVERVIEW

Disaster Planning Types

1. Strategic
2. Preparedness
3. Operations
   a. Security
   b. Communications
   c. Transport
   d. Staff health
   e. Beneficiary programs
4. Contingency
5. Evaluation

Planning precursors

1. Situation/Context Analysis
2. Stakeholder Analysis—identify stakeholders, capacity, and vulnerability for all areas of the potential work environment
3. SWOT Analysis—strengths, weaknesses, opportunities, and threats
4. Force Field Analysis—forces at play
5. Director's Vision of Success*—how you know when you get there
   a. mission and goal(s)
   b. boundary conditions—consequences to be avoided

Planning steps

1. Priorities*
2. Assumptions and Constraints
3. Problem Tree—performs root cause analysis, then summarizes cause and effects in a problem tree
4. Objectives Tree—reformulates problems identified above into objectives that are desirable and achievable, then summarizes means and ends in an objectives tree
5. Feasibility Analysis—technical, administrative, political, economic, and developmental analysis; analysis of alternatives; impact analysis (positive and negative); strategy selection*
6. Project Map—shows hierarchal relationship between purpose, components, results, and activities
7. Logframe—summarizes how and why
8. Workplan (implementation schedule, resource schedule)—summarizes when, and with what resources
9. Cost Schedule* (budget)—summarizes planned expenditures
10. Monitoring and Evaluation Plan
11. Reports Schedule
12. SOPs
13. Contingency Plans

* items need director's guidance/feedback

Document 5.2
PROJECT PLAN OF ACTION

Date

Executive Summary

A. **Goals** (Agency Intent)

B. **Strategy, Objectives, and Expected Results**

I. **SITUATION / CONTEXT ANALYSIS**

A. **Disaster History**

B. **Sociopolitical and Cultural Context** (on health status, health care services, and interventions)

C. **Security Situation**

D. **Resources and Capacities Available**

E. **Roles and Influence of Major Stakeholders** (eg military, non-state actors)

F. **Health Services** (SWOT and Constraints)

G. **Disaster Expected Evolution** (lessons learned from past experience)

H. **Reason for Agency Assistance**

II. **GOALS** (Agency Priorities and Intent)

A. **Mission**

1. Goals
2. Beneficiaries
3. Geographic location
4. Timeframe

B. **Vision of End State**

C. **Boundary Conditions**

1. Key decisions
2. Antigoals (unwanted outcomes)

III. **ASSUMPTIONS AND CONSTRAINTS**

A. **Assumptions**

1. Security and socioeconomic assumptions
2. Epidemiological assumptions

3. Health resource assumptions
4. Donor assumptions

B. Constraints

IV. STRATEGY, OBJECTIVES, AND EXPECTED RESULTS

A. Principles

1. Comprehensive approach involving PPRR
   a. all-hazards
   b. human and animal health
2. Integrated approach involving prepared community
3. Build on existing platforms and investments
4. Coordinate and leverage resources with other donors and private sector
5. Focus on high yield activities in high risk areas

B. Strategy

1. Population targeted
2. Subsector goods and services provided
3. Health system levels of care supported/restored

C. Objectives (eg in communicable diseases)

1. Prepare for epidemics
2. Prevent and control vaccine-preventable illnesses
3. Prevent and control vector-borne illnesses
4. Intensify disease surveillance system

D. Expected Results

1. 80% of targeted population or facilities

V. **KEY ACTIVITIES AND PERFORMANCE INDICATORS** (Logframe or Plan of Action by Objective)

Activity	Indicators	Means of Verification	Verifier	Input Needed	Date Done
Objective 1					
Activity 1	•	•			
Activity 2	•	•			
Objective 2					
Activity 1	•	•			
Activity 2	•	•			

VI. PROGRAM DESCRIPTION

A. Implementation Plan

B. Monitoring and Evaluation

C. Transition or Exit Strategy

VII. OUTPUTS AND OUTCOMES

A. Outputs

B. Impacts and Outcomes

1. Environmental
2. Health
3. Socioeconomic
4. Political
5. Financial

C. Sustainability

D. Contingency Planning

VIII. ACTIVITY OVERSIGHT

A. Organization Executive Officers

B. Project External Advisory Panel

C. Project Leadership Team

D. Field Supervisors

E. Field Staff

IX. REPORTING

A. Resource Management

1. Human resources
2. Material resources
3. Financial resources

B. Other POA Deliverables

1. Operations research

C. Incident Reports

D. Unexpected Consequences

X. SCHEDULE (Gantt Table)

XI. BUDGET

XII. ABBREVIATIONS

XIII. TECHNICAL ANNEXES (in chronological order of development)

A. Situation / Context Analysis

1. Stakeholder analysis (organization, community, population)
   a. identification
   b. strengths and weaknesses
   c. implementation capacity
   d. vulnerability
   e. preparatory assistance needed
   f. linkages
2. SWOT analysis (strengths & weaknesses of your org; opportunities and threats of the environment)
3. Force field analysis (forces at play)

B. Goals (Agency Priorities and Intent)

C. Assumptions and Constraints

D. Problem Tree (root cause analysis)

E. Objectives Tree (means to ends)

F. Feasibility Analysis

1. Technical
2. Administrative
3. Political
4. Economic
5. Developmental
6. Impact (positive and negative)

G. Project Map

H. Logframe

I. Workplan

1. Implementation schedule
2. Resource schedule

J. Cost Schedule (budget)

K. Monitoring and Evaluation Plan

L. Reports Schedule (templates)

M. SOPs (if not covered by the safety and security plan)

N. Contingency Plans

1. Major staff sickness (eg pandemic flu)
2. Border shutdown

Document 5.3
LOGICAL FRAMEWORK DEFINITIONS AND PROCESS

logical framework approach—analytical, presentational, and management tool involving a four part process which culminates in the logical framework matrix (logframe)

- problem analysis
- stakeholder analysis
- objectives analysis
- options analysis

The process serves to:

- analyze the existing situation
- identify vested interests (pro and con)
- establish a logical hierarchy of means by which objectives will be reached
- identify potential risks
- establish how outputs and outcomes might best be monitored
- present a project summary in standard format

logical framework matrix (logframe)—product of the logical framework approach

- **goal**—sectoral or national development impact to which the project contributes (written in the infinitive)
- **objective/purpose**—developmental outcome expected at the end of the project to which all components contribute (written in the infinitive)
- **component of objective**—specific outcome of each project output/activity area achieved by delivering specific outputs (written in the infinitive); each component has its specific sectoral, institutional, or technical focus and is likely to be managed by different groups within the targeted institution
    - training program design and delivery
    - facilities upgrading
    - project management
- **results/outputs**—direct measurable results in goods and services of the project (written in future perfect eg something will have been produced)
- **activities**—tasks carried out to deliver the identified outputs (written in present tense)
- **indicators**—measures of progress toward project goal, measure of extent to which component objectives have been achieved, quantity and quality of outputs, timing of delivery; they are SMART
    - **s**pecific
    - **m**easurable
    - **a**chievable (under one's responsibility, authority, influence, and technical competence)
    - **r**elevant
    - **t**ime-bound

- **means of verification (MOVs)**
  - who will collect data
  - what source, where located
  - when and how often
  - how to collect the data
  - what format to record the data
- **assumptions**—future conditions affecting project success over which the project manager has no direct control eg price stabilization, rainfall, land reform, etc
  - assumption—a condition, stated positively, upon which the project is dependent for objectives to be achieved
  - risk—a condition, stated negatively, which may prevent objectives from being achieved
  - killer assumption—an assumption judged as highly likely to change and critically undermine the project; when so identified, the project ought to be abandoned or redesigned

Logframe structure and completion sequence:

Project Description	Indicators	MOVs	Assumptions
1. Goal	10. Indicators	11. MOVs	
2. Objectives	12. Indicators	13. MOVs	9. Assumptions
3. Components	14. Indicators	15. MOVs	8. Assumptions
4. Results/ Outputs	16. Indicators	17. MOVs	7. Assumptions
5. Activities	milestones per activity scheduled	periodic reports	6. Assumptions

Overall, a logframe is a matrix, a logic, and a grammar. It can be cumbersome for the uninitiated. Many organizations, including WHO, use a simplified form of logframe to facilitate field use. This simplified approach may rely on predetermined indicator libraries, activity lists by subsector, and activity-based budgets. A well-developed logframe should be the STARTING point for operational planning. Inputs—resources required to undertake activities and produce outputs—are typically not specified in logframes, but are ultimately required for operational plans. Inputs commonly include:

- personnel
- information
- materials
- property, plant, and equipment
- time
- money
- organizational inputs
- complementary inputs
- unmet needs

Example:

Project Description	Indicators	MOVs	Assumptions
Goal	reduction of infant and child mortality by 30%	routine reports baseline and follow-up surveys	regarding relevance of project to program goals
Objectives	zero cases of measles in a designated 12 month period	epidemiological surveillance	regarding impact of services
Components			
Results/Outputs	80% of defined target population immunized	survey	regarding conversion of activities into results
Activities/Services	immunization program	service records	regarding conversion of resources into activities

Document 5.4
LOGFRAME TEMPLATE

	Intervention Logic	Objectively Verifiable Indicators of Achievement	Sources and Means of Verification	Assumptions
Program Goal	•	•	•	•
Objective or Component	•	•	•	•
Objective or Component	•	•	•	•

Expected Results	**<u>Objective</u> 1** •	•	•	
Expected Results	**<u>Objective</u> 2** •	•	•	
Expected Results	**<u>Objective</u> 3** •	•	•	

Document 5.5
PROJECT MONITORING AND EVALUATION WORKSHEET

Project Name:

Lead Agency & Subs:

Location:

Donors & Funding:

Duration:

Project Purpose:

Target Groups:

Project key contacts:

-
-
-
-

Component Description:

Component/Sector	Beneficiary Population Size	Location Province/District	When Start

General Feasibility Issues Arising

Security

Staff

Stuff

Spending

Technical

Administrative

Political

Economic

Developmental

Project Management Issues

Ref #	Components, Outputs, and Activities	Achievements by Component	Problems and Constraints	Actions Taken or Required
	Component 1			
	Output 1			
	• Activity 1			
	• Activity 2			
	• Activity 3			
	Output 2			
	• Activity 1			
	• Activity 2			
	• Activity 3			
	Output 3			
	• Activity 1			
	• Activity 2			
	• Activity 3			
	Output 4			
	• Activity 1			
	• Activity 2			

Document 5.6
REMOTE MANAGEMENT WORKSHEET

I. DEFINITION (ICRC [1])

The withdrawal of senior international or national humanitarian managers from the location of the provision of assistance or other humanitarian action as an adaptation to insecurity or denied access.

- It causes deviation from 'normal' programming practice.
- Program quality and effectiveness may suffer—particularly in impartiality of beneficiary selection and accountability of results.
- It may entail risk transfer to local partners.
- It is a last-resort modality short of suspending operations.

II. RATIONALE

A. Key Questions (ECHO [2])

1. Is there an access problem due to insecurity?
   a. Are there significant access issues impairing the delivery of humanitarian assistance which the implementing partner cannot resolve?
   b. In the same geographic area, is there no other humanitarian organization (eligible for ECHO funding) with the required capacity and experience willing and able to to meet the desired humanitarian needs thru direct action?
   c. Does the proposed intervention undermine efforts to resolve the security/bureaucratic obstacles?
2. Does the proposed action include acceptance-building measures?
   NB Acceptance of impartial and independent humanitarian action by local government, communities, and non-state actors is the most effective way to mitigate security risks for humanitarian workers and gain access to vulnerable populations. Insightful stakeholder mapping and experienced access negotiators are keys to the process.
   a. Does the proposed action identify actors at local, provincial, or international level who can impact access in proposed geographic areas?
   b. Does the proposed action include steps to gain, regain, or maintain acceptance of neutral and independent humanitarian action?
3. Is there a direct life-saving action?
   NB In view of associated risks, remote management is only be justified when it directly saves lives or preserves crucial livelihoods. Preparedness, early recovery, R2D, and resilience actions do not qualify.

4. Can the action be implemented without risking the lives of those undertaking the work on the ground?

   NB When management staff cannot verify the quality of the intervention, transfer of risk to field staff or to another implementer is not acceptable.

   a. Implementing partner must provide clear evidence that all possible measure have been put in place to reduce the risks for local staff undertaking the action. Implementing partner must provide clear evidence that programs are designed and delivered in manner that does not negatively impact on the security of disaster-affected communities and beneficiaries.

5. What is the source of the needs assessment in a remotely managed action?

   a. Implementing partner must specify what sources of information were used to estimate needs.
   b. Data collected remotely in conflict-affected areas (thru local staff, external partners, aerial surveillance, etc) must be verified by direct sources (IDPs, traders community representatives, etc).

6. Are staff on the ground adequately qualified and trained to manage the action, and are the information systems in place to provide them with needed information?

   a. Management staff must always have updated information on field level implementation.
   b. Skill gaps (technical, analytic, managerial) in field staff must be identified and remedied thru training or other measures.

7. Are the monitoring arrangements adapted for remote management?

   NB Effective monitoring requires a minimum level of face-to-face contact between managers, field staff, and beneficiaries. When managers cannot go to field sites, it may be possible for some beneficiaries to travel to a sub-office location. If that is not possible, remote managers must seek face-to-face meetings with stakeholders from affected areas (eg community representatives, traditional authorities, or traders).

   NB Risks of remote management increase over time—needs assessments may be outdated; risks may be inaccurately assessed; managers may lose touch with the field situation. "The longer humanitarian organizations rely on remote management to deliver assistance…the greater the risk that aid will become less effective." [2]

   a. Is there a mechanism of direct contact between program managers and beneficiaries or other local stakeholders?
   b. Are 3rd party monitors engaged? If so, they must be external to the conflict.

B. Indirect Monitoring Methods

1. Debriefing between iNGO and local partner
2. Mobile and web-based communications technology enabling call centers to check on staff, supplies, and operations at remote sites (difficult where field comms at remote sites are not accessible, reliable, or secure)
3. Phone complaint and feedback mechanisms (allowing beneficiaries to comment on type of assistance, quality of assistance, allegations of corruption, etc)
4. Complaint boxes
5. Broadcasts about planned activities (generally not feasible in conflicted areas)
6. Photos or videos of commodity distribution or service delivery
7. Web-based remote monitoring (via geo-tagged photos posted online or sent by email)
8. GPS shipment tracking (barcoding of shipment, scanning at dispatch and receipt)
9. Remote sensing
10. Voucher reconciliation
11. Peer monitoring (triangulation thru discussion with organizations working in the same area)
12. 3rd party monitoring (private firm with skilled personnel paid by implementing partner)—increasingly seen as gold standard
13. Crowd sourcing (via SMS, internet, Facebook)

References

1. Donini A, Maxwell D. (2013). From face-to-face to face-to-screen: remote management, effectiveness and accountability of humanitarian action in insecure environments. *International Review of the Red Cross*, *95*(890), 383–413. https://doi.org/10.1017/S1816383114000265.
2. ECHO. (2015). *ECHO's approach to remote management*. Available from: http://dgecho-partners-helpdesk.eu/actions_implementation/remote_management/start.

6 Medical Coordination

Contents

Overview

This section provides guidance on medical coordination. Medical coordinators should possess the technical competence to render an informed opinion, the administrative authority to mobilize resources, and the organizational responsibility for outcomes. Health cluster coordination is a specific application of medical coordination which requires specialized training and tools. It is essential that host health authorities lead the process, and that it embraces local providers and NGOs. Local culture, practices, and beliefs must inform decisions made about health programs. One must be aware of the insidious cycle of foreign actors paid by foreign donors who intervene on behalf of foreign constituencies, and then use external criteria to judge the adequacy of their work.

This section focuses on medical coordinator meeting processes and work products. Medical coordination meetings are an opportunity for the Ministry of Health and medical coordinators to develop consensus on health sector priorities, practices, and accountability. At those meetings, principles of engagement are an excellent way to begin substantive discussions. The process evidences the ability of medical coordinators to develop consensus on non-controversial areas. Failure to do so augurs poorly for the evolution of

D. A. Bradt, C. M. Drummond, *Pocket Field Guide for Disaster Health Professionals*,
https://doi.org/10.1007/978-3-030-04801-3_6

the relief effort. Meetings should be decisional, not just informational. Work products encompass:

- Coordination
- Rapid epidemiological assessment
- Minimum standards
- Epidemic preparedness
- Communicable disease control
- Epidemiological surveillance
- Health policy and personnel
- Medical logistics

Document 6.1
MEDICAL COORDINATOR WORK PRODUCTS

I. COORDINATION

A. List of Agencies, NGOs	contact list
B. Host Health System	organigram, description
C. Area-activity Table (who-what-where)	matrix
D. Partnership in Health Facilities (DHO + local NGO + iNGO)	
E. Coordination Meetings	meetings calendar, minutes

II. RAPID EPIDEMIOLOGICAL ASSESSMENT

A. Access to Affected	geographic mapping
B. Methodology	**template**
C. Priority Populations (eg CMR >1, size >1 k)	agreement

III. MINIMUM STANDARDS

A. Environmental Health — **minimum standards**

1. Water supply
2. Food supply
3. Sanitation
4. Shelter
5. Vector control

B. Clinical Medicine

1. Delivery of health services	health systems catchments
2. Standardization of case management	
(a) case definitions	**guidelines**
(b) treatment protocols (disease specific)	**guidelines** (see EHK, ELK)
(c) essential drug lists	**national guidelines** (see EHK)
(d) uniform referral practices	process
(e) secondary prevention	guidelines

IV. EPIDEMIC PREPAREDNESS	
A. Case Definitions	**guidelines**
B. Case Management Guidelines for Communicable Diseases	**guidelines**
C. Outbreak Management Protocol	**guidelines** (see ELK)
1. Alert thresholds	**table**
2. Staff investigation	**forms**
3. Specimen collection	**guidelines**
4. Lab to culture	**table**
D. Sources of Relevant Vaccines	list
E. Resource Prepositioning	**cholera kits**
F. Public Information	**templates**
V. COMMUNICABLE DISEASE CONTROL	
A. Disease-specific	**guidelines** (see ELK)
VI. EPIDEMIOLOGICAL SURVEILLANCE	
A. Data Sources	camp logbook
B. Reporting Forms	**reporting forms**
C. Collection Methods	
D. Data Analysis	
E. Reporting	**weekly reports**
VII. HEALTH POLICY AND PERSONNEL	personnel credentialing
VIII. MEDICAL LOGISTICS	**process**

bold generally pre-existing
ELK emergency library kit
EHK emergency health kit

Document 6.2
HEALTH CLUSTER PRINCIPLES OF COORDINATION

1. Authority to work in [country] is conferred by the Government of [country] through the Ministry of Health.
2. [Lead agency] authority to coordinate organizations in the health sector is conferred by the Ministry of Health. [Lead agency] is requested to convene health coordination meetings to establish a periodic forum at which to discuss technical and programmatic health issues affecting NGO and UN agency delivery of health services in [country].
3. Participants agree to conform to health policies and procedures established by statute of the Government of [country] and regulation of the Ministry of Health.
4. Participants agree to support minimum standards of humanitarian assistance as disseminated by the Sphere Project.
5. Participants agree to adhere to the Code of Conduct as disseminated by the Sphere Project.
6. Participants agree to fully characterize their organization's health activities in [country] to enable development of a health intervenor database which optimizes resources by identifying service gaps and preventing duplication of services.
7. Participants agree to undertake health activities relying on organizational competence to serve local needs with [lead agency] acting to encourage and coordinate multi-party involvement.
8. Meeting agendas are intended to support and complement interactions currently underway between participants and [country] health authorities.
9. Meeting discussions are intended to be interactive, field-oriented, and practical. The approach to health issues will involve disseminating information, examining problems, appraising options, developing consensus, making decisions, and implementing remedies.
10. Meeting minutes will be written by [lead agency] and disseminated to focal points among participant organizations and [country] health authorities to evidence ongoing transparency and professionalism among colleagues in humanitarian health assistance.

Document 6.3
HEALTH CLUSTER MEETING AGENDA

I. INTRODUCTIONS

II. INFORMATION UPDATE

A. Health Authorities Overview

B. Cluster System Update

C. Epidemiological Surveillance

D. Sectoral Issues (integrate with subgroup reports as subgroups are established)

1. Security, protection, & safety
2. Environmental health
3. Public health services
   a. disease prevention—eg vaccination
   b. epidemic preparedness and outbreak response
   c. health promotion and protection
4. Health facilities and clinical services
   a. vulnerable groups and access to care
   b. delivery of clinical health services
5. Medical logistics
6. Health financing, cost recovery

III. DISCUSSION

A. Domain-specific (across multiple settings, eg vaccination campaign)

B. Setting-specific (across multiple sectors, eg staff unrest in one locality)

C. Provider-specific (problems with one agency)

IV. ACTIVITY PLANNING AND PRIORITIZATION

Document 6.4
HEALTH CLUSTER MEETING PROCESS
Initial Meeting

Distribute attendance sheet and contact list

Goal: cooperation—shared goals and information

Purpose: maintain and improve the health status of the population in [specify area]

Intro round robin:
Name, Organization (may limit to 1 spokesperson/organization) mandates/missions, resources/capabilities, areas of responsibility, perceived operational priorities

Discussion:
1. Round robin protocol
   Who—one representative to speak for the agency (technically qualified, administratively authorized, organizationally responsible)
   What—situation update, urgent and important issues
2. TOR for the group
3. SAGs & TWiGs
4. Critical issues of the day
5. Future meeting schedule

Follow-up:
Action steps
Establish next time and place

Clerical duties of Medical Coordinator

- **Collect attendance sheet and contact list**
- **Write running minutes of the meeting**
  Attendance
  Discussion point summary (with apologies by MC for any misunderstandings or omissions)
    Administrative issues
    Documentation distributed
    General health issues—prioritized for follow-up at next meeting
  Follow-up
- **Compile draft contact list**

Document 6.4
HEALTH CLUSTER MEETING PROCESS
Subsequent Meetings

Distribute attendance sheet and contact list

Distribute blank gap identification forms

Goal: coordination—shared tasks; collaboration—shared resources

Purpose: improve the health status of the population in [specify area]

Intro round robin:
Name, organization (may limit to 1 spokesperson/organization if too many present)

Discussion:
1. TOR for the group (amend/assent)
2. SAGs & TWiGs
3. Critical issues of the day
4. Agenda for the meeting based upon issues and interest areas (give major headings only)
    Introductions (especially for new persons)
    Announcements (lead governmental authority)
    Subsector updates including local epidemiology
    New issues (rumors and reports)
        critical issues which will explode within 24 hours or require action to prevent imminent death)—develop subsector interest groups based upon recurrent issues
        info gaps → arrangements for initial assessment
        service gaps → gap filling, special planning
    Matching stated needs to locally available resources (personnel, equipment, $)

Follow-up:
1. Action steps
2. Establish next time and place

Clerical duties
- **Collect attendance sheet, contact list, and gap identification forms**
- **Write running minutes of the meeting**
    Attendance
    Discussion point summary (apologies by MC for any misunderstandings or omissions)
        Administrative issues
        Documentation distributed

Health authority announcements
General health issues—prioritized for follow-up meeting
Subsector updates
Follow-up

- **Revise contact list**
- **Compile health sector area-activity matrix from gap identification forms**
- **Compile health sector status summary**

7 Technical Annexes

Contents

D. A. Bradt, C. M. Drummond, *Pocket Field Guide for Disaster Health Professionals*,
https://doi.org/10.1007/978-3-030-04801-3_7

Overview

This section provides guidance on technical issues in the health sector. The annexes contain compilations of frequently used reference information.

- Humanitarian programs—contains conceptual frameworks on global clusters, relief programs, humanitarian financing, and early recovery.
- Security sector—contains key definitions from the Rome Statute of the International Criminal Court
- Health sector—contains a broad range of core health technical information including environmental classification of water and excreta-related diseases, disease prevention measures, water treatment end points, anthropometric classifications, micronutrient deficiency states, management of chemical weapon exposures, and epi methods.
- Tropical medicine—contains clinical summaries of tropical infectious diseases with details on disease vector and host, clinical presentation, diagnostic lab tests, clinical epidemiology, and therapy.
- Epidemic preparedness and response—contains core principles of epidemic preparedness and response.
- Communicable disease control—contains an overview of selected communicable diseases of epidemic potential including diarrhea, influenza, malaria, measles, meningitis, and viral hemorrhagic fever.
- Diagnostic laboratory—contains guidance on lab specimen handling and testing.
- Acronyms—contains acronyms commonly used in disaster management and humanitarian assistance.

Document 7.1
HUMANITARIAN PROGRAMS

I. HUMANITARIAN ASSISTANCE VALUES AND GOALS

A. Core Values

1. Humanity
2. Impartiality
3. Neutrality
4. Independence

B. Goals

1. Save lives
2. Alleviate suffering
3. Reduce economic and social impact of disaster
4. Undertake principled humanitarian action
5. Provide integrated multi-sector assistance and protection to the most vulnerable
6. Maintain peace and security
7. Uphold law and order (host government)
8. Implement durable solutions (UNHCR)
   a. repatriation
   b. local integration
   c. resettlement
9. Mitigate hazards
10. Build back better
11. Support community resilience, social cohesion, and early recovery

II. GLOBAL CLUSTERS AND LEADS (IASC [1,2])

A. Technical Areas		
1. Nutrition		UNICEF
2. Health		WHO
3. Water/sanitation		UNICEF
4. Emergency shelter	IDPs from conflict	UNHCR
	disaster situations	IFRC
5. Food security		WFP/FAO
B. Cross-cutting Areas		
1. Camp coordination	IDPs from conflict	UNHCR
	disaster situations	IOM
2. Protection		UNHCR
3. Early recovery		UNDP
4. Education		UNICEF/SC
C. Common Service Areas		
1. Logistics		WFP
2. Emergency telecoms		WFP

III. SECTORS AND THEMES

A. Sectors

1. Coordination
2. Protection and Registration
3. Security and Demobilization
4. Logistics
5. Site Planning
6. Water and Sanitation
7. Food Aid
8. Agriculture
9. Non-food Aid (household support)
10. Shelter
11. Health
12. Rehabilitation
13. Education and Training
14. Economic Recovery and Community Development
15. Durable Solutions

B. Cross-cutting Themes (IASC)

1. Human Rights & Protection
2. Gender
3. HIV/AIDS
4. Environment

C. Themes Per Donor Grants Guidelines

1. Artisanal Production
2. Capacity Building/Training
3. Cash Distribution
4. Cash for Work
5. Children
6. Conflict Resolution
7. Gender Relations
8. HIV-AIDS
9. Host Communities
10. Host Government
11. IDPs
12. Information Systems
13. Infrastructure Rehabilitation
14. Livelihoods/Income Generation
15. Market Rehabilitation
16. Micro-Finance/Micro-Credit
17. Nomads/Pastoralists
18. Protection Mainstreaming
19. Returnees
20. Slavery/Trafficking
21. Vouchers

IV. RELIEF PROGRAMS

A. Programming Principles

1. Address identified needs in underserved areas
2. Encourage local participation
3. Integrate beneficiaries into program planning
4. Collaborate with all stakeholders
5. Coordinate with all implementing partners
6. Plan comprehensive approaches
7. Develop community-based programs
8. Make inter-sectoral linkages (sector-wide approaches)
9. Use existing resources
10. Leverage outside resources of donors and private sector
11. Build on existing platforms
12. Apply international best practices
13. Target vulnerable populations
14. Focus on high impact activities
15. Ensure equitable access to services
16. Provide assistance acceptable to beneficiaries
17. Implement with cultural sensitivity
18. Reduce the local burden of disease
19. Enhance capacities
20. Reduce vulnerabilities
21. Alleviate poverty
22. Avoid dependency
23. Foster sustainable development
24. Support governmental priorities
25. Operate cost-effectively, transparently, and accountably

B. Programming Approach

1. Prioritize a core package of life-saving interventions in geographically targeted areas
2. Support humanitarian protection throughout the response
3. Provide flexible programming that lets partners adapt to new demands in new areas
4. Adopt market-based modalities
5. Enhance the humanitarian architecture
6. Support livelihoods programming that complements live-saving assistance when safe to do so to
7. Support early recovery and transition to development

C. Keys to Emergency Relief (M Toole, Burnet Institute, Melbourne, Australia, unpublished)

1. Intervene early
2. Support, not undermine, community coping strategies
3. Prevent communities from migrating
4. Avoid establishing large refugee camps
5. Establish a health information system

6. Ensure resources provided do not further divide communities
7. Focus on disease prevention
8. Work through existing structures and institutions
9. Insist that women control the distribution of relief supplies
10. Ensure open communication and coordination

D. Implementation Mechanics

1. Reallocation of existing local & national resources
2. Revision/refinement of present (medical) practices
   a. use of essential drugs
   b. use of standardized case management
   c. replacement of dated practices
3. Financial assistance (critical funding)
4. Technical assistance (critical skills)
   a. complement donated goods
   b. support appropriate technology
   c. develop information systems
5. Material assistance (critical goods)
   a. essential drugs and vaccines
   b. consumable supplies
   c. other stated needs of health authorities
6. Direct service provision (substitution)
7. Coordination of external assistance
   NB cooperation = shared goals; coordination = shared tasks; collaboration = shared resources
   a. identification and registration of actors
   b. actor/area/activity (who/what/where) matrix
   c. gap analysis and priority setting
   d. establishment of rapid response mechanism
   e. gap filling via complementary inputs linking iNGOs & local NGOs to local health authorities
      (1) technical
      (2) material
      (3) financial
   f. identification of deliverables and timetables
   g. consolidated reporting and dissemination
      (1) group terms of reference
      (2) meeting minutes
      (3) epidemiology updates
      (4) health sitreps
      (5) component analysis
      (6) field documentation (toolkit) for new arrivals
8. Capacity building of host authorities
9. Civil society partnership and support
   a. organize community leaders
   b. encourage gender mainstreaming
   c. encourage privatization
   d. discourage entitlements
10. Advocacy
11. Transition to early recovery

E. Strategy for Livelihood/Economic Relief

1. Restore productive assets (supply side interventions)
   a. in-kind donations (eg food, seeds, tools, fishing nets, etc)
   b. types of community projects in food-for-assets programs
      (1) natural resources development
         (a) water harvesting
         (b) soil conservation
      (2) restoration of agri(aqua)culture potential
         (a) irrigation systems
         (b) seed systems
      (3) infrastructure rehabilitation
         (a) schools
         (b) market places
         (c) community granaries
         (d) warehouses
         (e) roads
         (f) bridges
      (4) diversification of livelihoods
         (a) training and experience sharing
2. Increase individual purchasing power
   a. cash distribution
   b. cash for work (cash for assets)
   c. vouchers
   d. micro-credit
   e. job fairs
   f. artisanal production
   g. livelihoods/income generation
3. Support market resumption
   a. market rehabilitation
   b. infrastructure rehabilitation
   c. micro-finance institutions

F. Strategy for Early Recovery

Goals—protect what's left (1 month), restore the system (6 months), improve the system (6 months)

1. Adopt systems approach
   a. health services
   b. health workforce
   c. medical logistics (drugs, vaccines, equipment, supplies, & technology)
   d. health information system
   e. health financing
   f. leadership & governance
2. Phase in assistance to beneficiaries
   a. technical assistance
   b. material assistance
      (1) food
      (2) non-food items

- c. financial assistance
  - (1) cash grants
  - (2) cash for work
  - (3) microfinance (loans)
  - (4) livelihood/income generation

3. Ensure responsible resource management
   - a. human resources management
     - (1) incident management command and control
     - (2) team structure and function
     - (3) staff selection
       - (a) internationals
       - (b) homologues
     - (4) field activities
       - (a) briefing
       - (b) meetings and reports
       - (c) debriefing
     - (5) operations support
       - (a) comms
       - (b) transport
       - (c) office
       - (d) food and lodging
     - (6) personal health maintenance and morale
   - b. material resources management
   - c. financial resources management
   - d. supervision
   - e. monitoring and evaluation
4. Scale up coverage of priority health interventions
5. Address bottlenecks of the disrupted health system (otherwise temporary solutions become permanent)
6. Protect essential public health infrastructures
7. Build capacity of local authorities with focus on sustainable systems
   - a. technical oversight—hiring of local experts
   - b. material assistance—production of key commodities
   - c. financial assistance
8. Provide incentives for host government
9. Support host country non-beneficiary population
10. Find new partners in the development community
11. Use health Sustainable Development Goals as targets for recovery activities
12. Seek opportunities and develop mechanisms for transition and phase out

G. Program Constraints and Failures

1. Programmatic constraints
   - a. staff
     - (1) western trained
     - (2) hospital-based
     - (3) resource intensive

        (4) technology dependent
        (5) procedurally oriented
        (6) invasive
        (7) monolingual
        (8) hazard naïve
    b. supervision
        (1) limited responsibility
        (2) limited authority
        (3) limited accountability
    c. projects
        (1) acute
        (2) curative
        (3) short-term
        (4) intermittent
    d. systems
        (1) inadequate security
        (2) weak rule of law
        (3) limited accountability framework
        (4) uncoordinated humanitarian action
2. Project feasibility constraints
    a. security
    b. political
    c. administrative
    d. logistical
    e. technical
    f. economic
    g. developmental
3. Hazard-specific constraints (complex emergencies)
    a. hostile armed elements
    b. limited access
    c. overburdened provincial services
    d. limited information on beneficiaries

V. SOCIETAL RESILIENCE (hazards + environment + infrastructure + institutions + livelihoods)

A. Comprehensive Disaster Risk Management

1. DRM/DRR (where risk = hazard x vulnerability; also likelihood x impact)
2. Hazard and vulnerability analysis
3. Hazard and structural mitigation (eg climate change adaptation plans)
4. Disaster plans
    a. all-hazard plans vs hazard-specific plans
    b. preparedness plans
    c. contingency plans
    d. evacuation plans
    e. repurposing plans

    f. business continuity plans
    g. recovery plans
    h. R2D considerations
5. Early warning/early action systems
6. Emergency operation centers
7. Emergency relief supply systems
8. Disaster simulation exercises, tabletops, drills

B. Political

1. Proactive legislation and policy (not reactive)
2. Clear non-overlapping mandates
3. Funding commitment to comprehensive disaster management
4. Vertical and horizontal linkages in policy implementation
5. Comprehensive approaches to ecosystem protection rather than fragmentation based upon political jurisdictions
6. Generic approaches to managing technical (best) practices, but local approaches to managing community vulnerabilities
7. Communication and cooperation enabled between public and private sector, national level and local communities, and individual jurisdictions

C. Socioeconomic

1. Environmental impact of population growth
2. Environmental impact of dominant practices in land use and key livelihood sectors—agriculture, mining, manufacturing, pastoralism, etc.
3. Environmental and economic impact of hazard-specific zones, damages, and losses on biodiversity, ecosystems, and communities
4. Poverty alleviation and economic diversification programs
5. Inclusiveness thru use of gender disaggregated data
6. Indigenous knowledge and contribution to DRR
7. (Re)insurance mechanisms

D. Institutional

1. Leadership training programs
2. Transparent resource management
3. Open redundant communication channels
4. Streamlined work flows (no waste)
5. Robust information management and information sharing
6. MEAL programs
7. Accountability frameworks
8. Inter-agency coordination
9. Partnership development

E. Environment and Infrastructure

1. Hazard zoning
2. Hazard and structural mitigation
3. Remote sensing and early warning systems
4. Preventive maintenance

F. Community Capacities and Vulnerabilities

1. Lifeline protection (key infrastructure assets and systems)
   NB food for assets (using food, cash, or vouchers) programs can help build physical assets listed below (see VA2)
   a. security
   b. communication
   c. transportation
   d. energy
   e. environmental health (eg water supply, food security, shelter and housing)
   f. public health (eg disease surveillance, primary prevention)
   g. health
      (1) safe hospitals program
   h. education to achieve a literate and informed public
   i. information and DRR technologies
2. Social protection and safety nets (focus on women, vulnerable groups)
3. Livelihood protection

VI. DEVELOPMENT PROGRAMS

A. Strategic Objectives (USAID Policy Framework for Bilateral Foreign Aid [3])

1. Promote transformational development
   Support far-reaching, fundamental changes in relatively stable developing countries, with emphasis on improvements in governance and institutions, human capacity, and economic structure, so that countries can sustain further economic and social progress without depending on foreign aid. Focus on those countries with significant need for assistance and with adequate (or better) commitment to ruling justly, promoting economic freedom, and investing in people.
2. Strengthen fragile states
   Reduce fragility and establish the foundation for development progress by supporting stabilization, reform, and capacity development in fragile states when and where U.S. assistance can make a significant difference.
3. Support strategic states
   Help achieve major U.S. foreign policy goals in specific countries of high priority from a strategic standpoint.

4. Provide humanitarian relief
   Help meet immediate human needs, save lives, and alleviate suffering in countries afflicted by violent conflict, crisis, natural disasters, or persistent dire poverty.
5. Address global issues
   HIV/AIDS, other infectious diseases, climate change, direct support for international trade agreements, and counter narcotics.

B. Approaches (USAID Gender Equality and Female Empowerment Policy [4])

1. Adopt inclusive approach
2. Integrate gender equality into all work
3. Build partnerships
4. Harness science, technology, and innovation
5. Address unique challenges in crises and conflict-affected communities
6. Serve as thought leader
7. Be accountable

C. Partnership Mechanisms (US National Strategy for Pandemic Influenza [5])

1. International cooperation to protect lives and health
2. Timely and sustained high-level political leadership to the disease
3. Transparency in reporting of cases of disease in humans and in animals caused by strains that have pandemic potential to increase understanding, enhance preparedness, and ensure rapid and timely response to potential outbreaks
4. Immediate sharing of epidemiological data and clinical samples with the World Health Organization (WHO) and the international community to characterize the nature and evolution of any outbreaks as quickly as possible
5. Prevention and containment of an incipient epidemic through capacity building and in-country collaboration with international partners
6. Rapid response to the first signs of accelerated disease transmission
7. Work in a manner supportive of key multilateral organizations (WHO, FAO, OIE)
8. Timely coordination of bilateral and multilateral resource allocations; dedication of domestic resources (human and financial); improvements in public awareness; and development of economic and trade contingency plans
9. Increased coordination and harmonization of preparedness, prevention, response and containment activities among nations
10. Actions based on the best available science

D. Program Innovations at Community Level

1. Community interventions
   a. sector-wide approaches (SWAps)
   b. integrated health interventions
      (1) PHC
      (2) SPHC
      (3) IMCI
   c. home-based interventions
      (1) CTC
   d. microfinance
      (1) Grameen Bank
2. Best practice program models (centers of excellence arising within a community)
   a. Matlab Health Research Center (part of ICDDR, Bangladesh)
   b. Shoklo Malaria Research Unit, Tak Province, Thailand
   c. Fistula Hospital, Addis Ababa, Ethiopia
   d. Behrhorst Clinic, Guatemala
3. Self-replicating centers of excellence
   a. Fistula Hospital, Addis Ababa, Ethiopia

VII. SEEDS OF CHANGE

A. Innovators

B. Thought Leaders

C. Change Agents and Influencers

D. Early Adopters

E. Craft Groups

F. Centers of Excellence

G. Communities of Practice

H. Global Alliance

I. Crowds

References

1. Inter-agency Standing Committee. Guidance Note on Using the Cluster Approach to Strengthen Humanitarian Response. November 24, 2006. Available from: https://interagencystandingcommittee.org/system/files/legacy_files/Cluster%20implementation%2C%20Guidance%20Note%2C%20WG66%2C%2020061115-.pdf.
2. OCHA. Global Cluster Leads (as of June 2012). Available from: http://reliefweb.int/sites/reliefweb.int/files/resources/map_2809.pdf.

3. USAID. Policy framework for bilateral foreign aid. January 2006. Available from USAID's Development Experience Clearinghouse https://www.dec.usaid.gov, and https://www.usaid.gov/sites/default/files/documents/1868/201mam.pdf.
4. USAID. Gender equality and female empowerment policy. March 2012. Available from: https://www.usaid.gov/sites/default/files/documents/1865/GenderEqualityPolicy_0.pdf.
5. US Homeland Security Council. National strategy for pandemic influenza. November 2005. Available from: http://www.flu.gov/planning-preparedness/federal/pandemic-influenza.pdf.

Document 7.2
SECURITY SECTOR

I. DEFINITIONS (Rome Statute [1])

A. Crimes (within the International Criminal Court's Jurisdiction) (Article 5)

1. Genocide (Article 6)—acts committed with intent to destroy, in whole or in part, a national, ethnic, racial, or religious group
   a. killing members of the group
   b. causing serious bodily or mental harm to members of the group
   c. inflicting on the group conditions of life calculated to bring about its physical destruction in whole or in part
   d. imposing measures intended to prevent births within the group
   e. forcibly transferring children of the group to another group
2. Crimes against humanity (Article 7)—acts committed as part of a widespread or systematic attack against any civilian population, with knowledge of the attack
   a. murder
   b. extermination
   c. enslavement
   d. deportation
   e. imprisonment in violation of international law
   f. torture
   g. rape, sexual slavery, enforced prostitution, forced pregnancy, enforced sterilization, or other comparable form of sexual violence
   h. persecution on political, racial, national, ethnic, cultural, religious, gender, or other grounds universally recognized as impermissible under international law
   i. enforced disappearance
   j. apartheid
   k. other inhumane acts intentionally causing great suffering or serious injury to body or to mental or physical health
3. War crimes (Article 8)
   a. grave breaches of the Geneva Conventions of 12 Aug 1949
      (1) willful killing
      (2) torture or inhumane treatment including biological experiments
      (3) willfully causing great suffering
      (4) extensive destruction and appropriation of property
      (5) compelling a POW to serve in the armed forces of a hostile power
      (6) willfully depriving a POW of the right to a fair trial
      (7) unlawful deportation
      (8) taking of hostages

b. serious violations of laws and customs applicable in international armed conflict
   (1) intentionally directing attacks against the civilian population or against civilians not taking direct part in hostilities
   (2) intentionally directing attacks against civilian objects
   (3) intentionally directing attacks against personnel, installations, material, units, or vehicles involved in humanitarian assistance or peacekeeping mission
   (4) intentionally launching an attack in the knowledge that it will cause incidental civilian loss of life or severe damage to the natural environment
   (5) attacking undefended towns, villages, dwellings, or buildings which are not military targets
   (6) killing or wounding a combatant who has surrendered
   (7) improper use of a flag of truce, flag or insignia or uniform of the enemy or of the UN, or emblems of the Geneva conventions resulting in death or serious personal injury
   (8) transfer by the Occupying Power of parts of its own civilian population into the territory it occupies, or the deportation or transfer of all or parts of the population of the occupied territory within or outside the territory
   (9) intentionally directing attacks against buildings dedicated to religion, education, art, science, charitable purposes, historic monuments, hospitals, and places where sick are collected, provided they are not military objectives
   (10) subjecting persons to physical mutilation or to medical or scientific experiments which are not justified by the medical treatment nor carried out in his/her interest
   (11) killing or wounding treacherously individuals belonging to the hostile nation or army
   (12) declaring that no quarter will be given
   (13) destroying or seizing the enemy's property unless such be imperatively demanded by the necessities of war
   (14) declaring abolished, suspended, or inadmissible in a court of law the rights and actions of the nationals of the hostile party
   (15) compelling the nationals of the hostile party to take part in the operations of war directed against their own country
   (16) pillaging a town or place, even when taken by assault
   (17) employing poison or poison weapons
   (18) employing asphyxiating, poisonous or other gases, and all analogous liquids, materials, or devices

(19) employing bullets which expand or flatten easily in the human body
(20) employing weapons, projectiles, material and methods of warfare which cause superfluous injury or unnecessary suffering
(21) committing outrages upon personal dignity, in particular humiliating and degrading treatment
(22) committing rape, sexual slavery, enforced prostitution, forced pregnancy, enforced sterilization, or other comparable form of sexual violence
(23) utilizing a civilian or other protected person to render certain areas or military forces immune from military operations
(24) intentionally directing attacks against buildings, material, medical units, transport, and personnel using the emblems of the Geneva Conventions in conformity with international law
(25) conscripting or enlisting children under the age of 15 years

c. serious violations of common article 3 applicable in non-international armed conflict, ie acts vs persons taking no active part in the hostilities, including armed forces placed hors de combat by sickness, wounds, detention, or other cause
   (1) violence to life and person
   (2) outrages upon personal dignity
   (3) taking of hostages
   (4) passing of sentences and carrying out of executions
d. non-applicability of c to internal disturbances (riots, sporadic violence, etc)
e. other serious violations of laws and customs applicable in non-international armed conflict (gen // 3b above)

4. Crime of aggression (provision to be adopted)

II. ARMED PERPETRATORS

A. Regular Military (enlisted or conscripted)
B. Militias
C. Mercenaries
D. Ethnic and Religious Extremists
E. Affiliates of A-D
F. Rogue Elements and Dissidents
G. Peacekeeping Forces
H. Organized Criminals
I. Petty Criminals

III. HEALTH CONSEQUENCES OF SECURITY BREAKDOWN

A. Decreased Access and Protection for Beneficiaries

1. Besieged areas
2. Lawlessness

3. Forced displacement
4. Decreased access to lifeline systems (water, sanitation, food, power, communications) thru destruction, roadblocks, curfews, discrimination
5. Decreased access to humanitarian assistance as above
6. Discrimination and persecution
   a. age
   b. gender
   c. race
   d. religion
   e. ethnicity
   f. geographic origin
   g. political affiliation
   h. socioeconomic status
   i. sexual orientation
   j. HIV status
   k. disability status
   l. migratory status

B. Increased Morbidity and Mortality

1. Direct trauma—death, injury, disability, murder, mutilations, torture, SGBV, psychosocial suffering
2. Diseases of overcrowding and displacement
3. Outbreaks of preventable and previously controlled diseases
4. Untreated chronic illnesses
5. Morbidity & mortality multipliers (measles, malnutrition, TB/HIV)
6. High risk behavior to address basic needs
   a. exposure to military conflict and ordnance
   b. criminality
   c. transactional/survival sex
   d. child exploitation

C. Degradation of Health System

1. Damage/destruction of health facilities and critical infrastructure
2. Degradation/disruption of health services complicated by increased demand from population influxes and decreased access to care
3. Threats to, attacks on, and attrition of health personnel
4. Disruption of medical logistics
5. Disruption of health information systems and telecommunications at large
6. Under-resourced health financing
7. Weak health governance

D. Loss of Human Capital and Physical Assets

E. Loss of Development Opportunity for Society

IV. SECURITY STEPS TO INITIATING SERVICES IN CONFLICT ZONES

A. Identification of Ground Contacts and Formation of Security Network

B. Initiation of UNHAS Flights

C. Initiation of Day Missions

1. security detail on team with comms equipment and plan
2. contingency packs with tent, sleeping bags, and water in case of security breakdown
3. ground situation to be ascertained before mission departure

D. Establishment of Humanitarian Hub

V. SECURITY OBJECTIVES

A. Unimpeded Access to Beneficiaries

1. Registration/verification
2. Protection
3. Humanitarian assistance
4. Family reunification
5. Information dissemination

B. Security for Refugees and Humanitarian Personnel

1. MOSS and SOPs
2. Security Focal Points
3. Security Ops Center with daily briefings
4. Cessation of hostilities
5. DDRRR
6. Peace agreements

C. Law Enforcement

1. Appropriate civil authorities
2. Search for accountability
3. Perpetrators of violence are arrested, charged, and tried in a civil court of law

D. Free and Informed Choices

E. Program Participation of Beneficiaries (especially women)

F. Relocation (only if voluntary, people are medically fit, and families are united)

Reference

1. Rome Statute of the International Criminal Court, July 17, 1998, 2187 U.N.T.S. 90. Available from: http://untreaty.un.org/cod/icc/statute/romefra.htm.

Document 7.3
HEALTH SECTOR

Glossary

ABX	antibiotics
AFP	acute flaccid paralysis
AIDS	acquired immune deficiency syndrome
ASDR	age-specific death rate
BCG	bacillus Calmette-Guérin
BMI	body mass index
c	with
cc	cubic centimeter
CDR	crude death rate
CFR	case fatality ratio
CI	confidence interval
cm	centimeter
CMAM	community-based management of acute malnutrition
CSS	cluster sample survey
CTC	community therapeutic care (malnutrition management)
d	day
D5	dextrose 5% in water
D10	dextrose 10% in water
D&C	dilation and curettage
D_{eff}	design effect
DTP	diphtheria + tetanus + pertussis vaccine
DRR	disaster risk reduction
EOC	Emergency Operations Center
EPI	Expanded Programme on Immunization
gm	gram
GAM	global acute malnutrition
gtt	drops
h	hour
H	height
HAM	height-for-age median
HAZ	height-for-age z score
HB	hepatitis B
HCW	health care worker
HH	household
Hib	*Haemophilus influenzae* type b
HIV	human immunodeficiency virus
ICDDR	International Centre for Diarrhoeal Disease Research, Bangladesh
ICS	incident command system
ID	infectious disease
IMCI	Integrated Management of Childhood Illness (WHO initiative)

IMPAC	Integrated Management of Pregnancy and Childbirth (WHO initiative)
IMR	infant mortality rate
IPD	inpatient department
IV	intravenous
kg	kilogram
L	liter
L&D	labor and delivery
m	meter
MAM	moderate acute malnutrition
MCI	mass casualty incident
MCV	measles-containing vaccine
MD	medical doctor
mg	milligram
MISP	Minimum Initial Service Package (used in reproductive health)
mL	milliliter
MMR	measles + mumps + rubella vaccine
mo	month
MR	measles + rubella vaccine
MSF	Médecins sans Frontières
MUAC	mid-upper arm circumference
NGO	non-governmental organization
NGT	nasogastric tube
NID	national immunization day(s)
NL	normal
NS	normal saline
O10	over 10 year-old
OPD	outpatient department
OPV	oral polio vaccine
OR	operating room
ORS	oral rehydration solution
OTP	outpatient therapeutic program
PCV	pneumococcal conjugate vaccine
PLW	pregnant and lactating women
PO	by mouth
ppm	parts per million
RL	Ringer's lactate
RUSF	ready-to-use supplementary food
RUTF	ready-to-use therapeutic food
RV	rotavirus
Rx	medication
SAM	severe acute malnutrition
SC	stabilization center
SD	standard deviation
SFC	supplementary feeding center
SFP	supplementary feeding program

SIA	supplemental immunization activities
SOP	standard operating procedure
t	teaspoon
T	tablespoon
TB	tuberculosis
TFC	therapeutic feeding center
Tx	treatment
U5	under 5 year-old
U5DR	under 5 year-old death rate
U5MR	under 5 year-old mortality rate
U10	under 10 year-old
W	weight
WASH	water, sanitation, and hygiene
W/H	weight-for-height
WHM	weight-for-height median
WHO	World Health Organization
WHZ	weight-for-height z score
wk	week
YF	yellow fever
yr	year

I. CORE DISCIPLINES IN DISASTER HEALTH

A. Clinical Medicine

1. Prehospital care
2. Primary, preventive, and basic services
   a. comprehensive primary health care
   b. child health services
   c. reproductive health services
   d. trauma services
   e. mental health services
   f. chronic diseases
   g. infection control
3. Referral care

B. Public Health

1. Rapid epidemiological assessment (minimum essential data sets)
2. Inter-agency health coordination
3. Standardized case management
4. Environmental health (minimum standards)
5. Epidemic preparedness and response
6. Disease surveillance (surveillance case definitions, data flow, and analysis)
7. Special surveys (cluster sample surveys)
8. Health policy and personnel planning
9. Immunization programs (EPI)
10. Medical logistics

C. Disaster Management

1. Site security
2. Urban search and rescue
3. Hazard-specific issues (hazard analysis, mitigation, decontamination, vulnerability reduction)
4. Disaster response modalities (ICS/EOC)
5. Geographic information systems
6. Public information
7. Community recovery

D. WHO Mandated Responsibilities in Disaster

1. Core functions (World Health Assembly Res 58.1)
   a. needs assessment
   b. health coordination
   c. gap filling
   d. capacity building
   NB protection & nutrition are beyond the mandate of WHO

2. Critical functions in emergency response (WHO *Emergency Response Framework*)
   a. leadership
   b. information
   c. technical expertise
   d. core services

II. PRIMARY HEALTH CARE PROGRAMS

A. Primary Health Care (Declaration of Alma Ata [1])

1. Health education
2. Food and nutrition
3. Water and sanitation
4. Maternal and child health, family planning
5. Immunization
6. Prevention of endemic disease
7. Treatment of common disease and injury
8. Essential drugs

B. Selective Primary Health Care (Walsh and Warren [2])

1. Growth monitoring
2. Oral rehydration therapy
3. Breast feeding
4. Immunization
5. Female literacy
6. Family planning
7. Food supplements

III. DISEASE PREVENTION

A. Definitions

1. Primary (individual without disease)
   Goal—prevent the disease from starting (consider host-agent-environment)
   a. limit pathogenesis of a disease-causing agent (eg lower cholesterol levels)
   b. alter the environment to keep the disease from humans (eg regulate asbestos exposures)
   c. strengthen host resistance to the disease (eg measles immunization, water fluoridation)
2. Secondary (individual with disease but without symptoms)
   Goal—prevent disease symptoms and complications from developing
   a. intervene after exposure (eg rabies vaccination)
   b. detect and treat disease before it becomes symptomatic (eg cancer screening)

c. prevent disease spread by treating contacts (eg TB exposure treatment)

3. Tertiary (individual with symptomatic disease)
   Goal—cure or control of clinical disease (bulk of clinical medicine)
   a. cure disease or reverse clinical manifestations (eg appendectomy, thrombolysis)
   b. control disease progression to avoid complications (eg retroviral drugs, anticoagulation in atrial fibrillation)
   c. control spread of disease to others (eg TB case management)

B. **Vaccinations**

1. Infant schedule (WHO)

Table 7.3.1
Infant Vaccination Schedule

Age	Vaccine
Birth	BCG, HB-1, ± OPV birth dose
6 wks	DTP-1, OPV/IPV-1, HB-2, Hib-1, PCV-1, RV-1
10 wks	DTP-2, OPV/IPV-2, HB-3, Hib- 2, PCV-2, RV-2
14 wks	DTP-3, OPV/IPV-3, HB-4, Hib-3, PCV-3, RV-3
9–12 mo	MCV-1 (eg MR or MMR)
15 mo	MCV-2

NB Table does not convey all options for vaccine administration. Diphtheria toxoid is not manufactured as monovalent vaccine. It is combined with tetanus toxoid—either full-strength dose for pediatric use (DT), or reduced-strength dose for adult use (Td). These are combined with acellular or whole-cell pertussis antigens—either full-strength dose for pediatric use (DTaP, DTwP), or reduced-strength dose for adolescent/adult use (Tdap).

DTP-1 is a good indicator of access to care.

DTP-3 is a good indicator of ultimate service delivery.

2. Immunization program

Table 7.3.2
Immunization Program Components

Intervention	Polio	Measles
Routine immunization	+	+
Supplementary immunization	National immunization days (NID)	Supplementary immunization activities (SIA)
Surveillance	Acute flaccid paralysis (AFP)	Case-based
Case follow-up	Mop-up campaign	Case management

3. Vaccine quantities

Table 7.3.3
Calculation of Vaccine Quantities

Indicator & benchmark	Quantity
Total population	100,000
Target population (6 mo – 15 yr) 45% total	45,000
Cover objective = 100%	45,000
Number of doses (1 for measles)	45,000
Expected loss 15%	52,940
Increase reserve by 25%	66,175
Round up	67,000

IV. CLINICAL FACILITIES

A. Generic Profile

	Fixed Clinics	Health Centers	District Hosp
1. Quantity			
2. Catchment population	5–10 k	< 50 k	100 k
3. Access to facility	self	self	referral
4. Staffing			
a. quantity (~1/1000 p)	2–5 staff	5–10 staff	variable
b. skill mix	1 HCW	5 HCW, 1 MD	5 MD, 1 surgeon
5. Caseload (% of catchment population/d)	1–10%	1–10%	
6. Bed capacity (10/10,000 population)			
7. Bed occupancy			
8. Referral load (% of caseload)	10%	10%	
9. Referral system			
10. Clinical services	OPD, ORS	+ IPD, L&D	+ OR

a. departments/units (verify functioning of expected services)			
(1) clinical			
(a) OPD	+	+	+
(b) IPD	–	+	+
(c) L&D	–	+	+
(d) surgery	–	+/–	+
(e) other			
(2) dispensary	+/–	+	+
(3) diagnostic lab	+/–	+	+
(4) blood bank	–	–	+
(5) radiology	–	–	+

V. REPRODUCTIVE HEALTH

A. Safe Motherhood (IMPAC, MISP)

NB 15% of pregnant women have complications requiring emergency OB care; 5% (3–7%) need C-section; 10% of deliveries will have primary post-partum hemorrhage within 24 h

1. Causes of maternal death — Time to death
   a. other emergencies 22% — ruptured uterus—1 d
   b. hemorrhage 18% — ante-partum—12 h, post-partum—2 h
   c. eclampsia 12% — 2 d
   d. obstructed labor 8% — 3 d
   e. sepsis 9% — 6 d
   f. unsafe abortion 18% — variable
   g. other indirect (malaria, HIV) 13% — variable
2. Basic emergency obstetric care (1 facility/125 k pop)
   a. parenteral antibiotics
   b. parenteral oxytocics
   c. parenteral anticonvulsants for pre-eclampsia & eclampsia
   d. manual removal of placenta
   e. removal of retained products (vacuum aspiration, D&C)
   f. assisted vaginal delivery (vacuum, forceps)
3. Comprehensive emergency obstetric care (as above plus below) (1 facility/500 k pop)
   a. Caesarean section (5–15% of deliveries)
   b. blood transfusion
4. Treatment of obstructed labor
   a. McRoberts maneuver—flex thighs at the hips and push knees to maternal abdomen
   b. pressure on suprapubic area
   c. proctoepisiotomy
   d. Wood's corkscrew maneuver—rotate shoulders 180° or to an oblique diameter to disengage the impacted shoulder
   e. delivery of the posterior arm (> incidence of humerus and clavicle fractures)

f. symphysiotomy
g. Zavanelli maneuver—replace head into the vagina and perform C-section

5. Essential newborn care
   a. basic newborn resuscitation
   b. warmth (drying and kangaroo care)
   c. eye prophylaxis (tetracycline ointment)
   d. clean cord care
   e. early and exclusive breast feeding
6. Delays to care
   a. delay in deciding to seek care
   b. delay in reaching care
   c. delay in receiving adequate care

VI. WATER AND SANITATION

A. Classification (D Mara, R Feachem [3])

Table 7.3.4
Environmental Classification of Water & Excreta Related Diseases

Diseases	Pathogen/disease	Preventive Measures
Fecal-oral = water-borne + water-washed	Virus—hepatitis A/E, polio, rotavirus, adenovirus	Water-washed: > H_2O quantity Water-borne: > H_2O quality
	Bacteria—*Campylobacter, E. coli, Salmonella, Shigella, Vibrio*	
	Protozoa—*Entamoeba, Balantidium, Cryptosporidium, Giardia, Isospora*	
	Helminths—*Ascaris, Enterobius*	
Non-fecal-oral water-washed	Skin infections—scabies, leprosy, yaws	> H_2O quantity; > Hygiene education
	Eye infections—trachoma, conjunctivitis	
	Louse-borne fevers	

Diseases	Pathogen/disease	Preventive Measures
Water-based	Bacteria—*Leptospira, Francisella, Legionella*	< Contact with contaminated H_2O
	Helminths—*Schistosoma, Clonorchis, Fasciola, Paragonimus, Dracunculus*	
Insect-vectored, water-related Mosquitoes (breeding in water), flies (biting/ breeding near water)	Malaria, dengue, Rift Valley fever, Japanese encephalitis, yellow fever, sleeping sickness, oncho, filariasis	Destroy breeding sites; Use barrier precautions (ITNs)
Insect-vectored, excreta-related Flies, cockroaches	Includes all fecal-oral diseases + water-based helminths + geohelminths + taeniasis	> Environmental hygiene
Rodent-vectored	Similar to insect-vectored, excreta-related but includes all water-based pathogens listed (except *Legionella*)	> Rodent control; < Contact with contaminated H_2O
Geohelminths	Roundworm, hookworm, whipworm	Excreta disposal
Taenia	Beef and pork tapeworm	Excreta disposal; Proper meat cooking

Source: D Mara, R Feachem in *Journal of Environmental Engineering* © 1999. Used with permission of ASCE.

B. Prevention (adapted from R Feachem [4])

Table 7.3.5
Water & Excreta Related Disease Prevention Measures

Disease	Prevention Measures						
	H_2O quality	H_2O quantity	Excreta disposal	Excreta Tx	Personal hygiene	Waste H_2O disposal	Food hygiene
Diarrheal disease & enteric fevers							
Viral	2	2	1	1	2	0	1
Bacterial	3	3	2	1	3	0	3
Protozoal	1	3	2	1	3	0	2
Polio, Hepatitis A	1	3	2	1	3	0	1
Water-washed (skin, eye, louse-borne disease)	0	3	0	0	3	0	0
Water-based							
Schisto	1	1	3	2	1	0	0
Guinea worm	3	0	0	0	0	0	0
Clonorchis	0	0	2	2	0	0	3
Water-related							
Malaria	0	0	0	0	0	1	0
Dengue, YF	0	0	0	0	0	1	0
Filariasis	0	0	3	0	0	3	0
Worms without intermediate host	0	1	3	2	1	0–1	1–2
Worms with intermediate host	0	0	3	3	0	0	3

Source: R Feachem in *Water Supply and Sanitation in Developing Countries* © 1983. Used with permission of Chartered Institution of Water and Environmental Management.
0 = no importance; 3 = great importance

A range of generic prevention measures should be considered for its impact on diseases in a biological "all-hazards" environment. Overall, excreta disposal, water quantity, personal hygiene, and food hygiene commonly contribute more to environmental health than do other listed measures. Epidemic threats will oblige heightened consideration of disease-specific strategies for prevention and control.

C. Water Treatment (bold text of particular relevance in clinical facilities)

1 ppm = 1 mg/kg (solids)
= 1 mg/L (liquids) = 1 ug/mL (liquids) = basic unit of measure for chloroscopes
:10,000 ppm = 1%

Table 7.3.6
Chlorine Concentration and Uses

PPM	Equivalents	Concentration %	Use
0.5	0.5 mg/L 0.0005 gm/L,mg/mL 0.00005 gm/100 mL	0.00005%	Piped water systems, goal for all end user drinking water
1	1 mg/L 0.001 gm/L, mg/mL 0.0001 gm/100 mL	0.0001%	Standpost systems
2	2 mg/L 0.002 gm/L, mg/mL 0.0002 gm/100 mL	0.0002%	Pre-treatment for selected/ known water sources—tanker trucks at filling stations, protected tube wells, clear rainwater
5	5 mg/L 0.005 gm/L, mg/mL 0.0005 gm/100 mL	0.0005%	Pre-treatment for untested/ unknown water sources—unprotected wells, cloudy surface water; filter/flocculate before chlorinating
10	10 mg/L 0.01 gm/L, mg/ mL 0.001 gm/100 mL	0.001%	Water with known fecal contamination; filter/flocculate before chlorinating
30	30 mg/L .03 gm/L, mg/mL .003 gm/100 mL	0.003%	Water from contaminated well or borehole (needs super-chlorination to achieve breakpoint chlorination)
50	50 mg/L 0.05 gm/L, mg/ mL 0.005 gm/100 mL	0.005%	Utensil rinse in restaurants (USA)

PPM	Equivalents	Concentration %	Use
500	**500 mg/L 0.5 gm/L, mg/mL 0.05 gm/100 mL**	**0.05%**	**Hands, skin (eg wash points)**
2000	**2000 mg/L 2 gm/L, mg/mL 0.2 gm/100 mL**	**0.2% (0.5% at ICDDR)**	**Cholera cots, covers, floors, walls, equipment, clothing, isolation areas (cholera, dysentery, influenza epidemics)**
10,000	10,000 mg/L 10 gm/L, mg/mL 1 gm/100 mL	1%	Latrine door handles
20,000	**20,000 mg/L 20 gm/L, mg/mL 2 gm/100 mL**	**2%**	**Body fluids (stool, vomitus)—stool buckets, corpses (disinfection for burial), shoes (perimeter control)**
50,000	50,000 mg/L 50 gm/L, mg/mL 5 gm/100 mL	5%	Household bleach

Table 7.3.7
Chlorine Products and Dilution

Product	Potable water treatment 0.0005%	Hands and skin cleaning 0.05%	Bedding/ clothes cleaning 0.5%	Body fluid/ corpse cleaning 2.0%
Household bleach Sodium hypochlorite solution 5% active chlorine (50 mg/mL)	2.5 mL in 5 gal ≈ 8 gtt/gal, 2 gtt/L ≈ 6 mg/L or 6 PPM NB double if source is contaminated	100 mL in 10 L water	1 liter in 10 L water	4 liters in 6 L water
Bleaching powder Chlorinated lime 30% active chlorine		16 g (1 T) to 10 L water	16 g (1 T) to 1 L water	64 g (4 T) to 1 L water

Product	Potable water treatment 0.0005%	Hands and skin cleaning 0.05%	Bedding/ clothes cleaning 0.5%	Body fluid/ corpse cleaning 2.0%
High-test hypochlorite (HTH) Calcium hypochlorite Chlorine granules 70% active chlorine		7 g (0.5 T) to 10 L water	7 g (0.5 T) to 1 L water	28 g (2 T) to 1 L water

VII. FOOD AND NUTRITION

Malnutrition is #1 risk to child health worldwide. It contributes to an estimated 2.5 M out of 6.3 M U5 deaths/year.

A. Prediction and Early Warning Systems

1. FEWS NET products
   a. Food Security Outlook (FSO)—assumptions and 8-mo projections issued 3x/year
   b. Food Security Outlook Update (FSOU)—update mid-term between FSOs
   c. Key Messages (KM)—precedes FSO
   d. Price Bulletin (PB)
   e. Food Assistance Outlook Brief (FAOB)—regional outlook
2. FEWS NET distribution calendar
   a. January – Key Messages (KM)
   b. **February – Food Security Outlook (FSO)**
   c. March – Key Messages (KM)
   d. April – Food Security Outlook Update (FSOU)
   e. May – Key Messages (KM)
   f. **June – Food Security Outlook (FSO)**
   g. July – Key Messages (KM)
   h. August – Food Security Outlook Update (FSOU)
   i. September – Key Messages (KM)
   j. **October – Food Security Outlook (FSO)**
   k. November – Key Messages (KM)
   l. December – Food Security Outlook Update (FSOU) (optional)

B. Protein-calorie Malnutrition

1. Screening
   U5—mid-upper arm circumference (MUAC) used as a screening tool in pedes and adults. In pedes, < 13.5 cm or edema is referred for W/H measurements.

2. Individual diagnosis
   a. pedes (U10)anthropometrics: ΔW/H before ΔW/Age before ΔH/Age

Acute <-> Chronic

Table 7.3.8
Anthropometric Indicators in Children

Combined anthropometrics		**W/H % of median**	
		> 80% (NL)	< 80%
H/Age % of median	> 90% (NL)	NL	Wasted
	< 90%	Stunted	Wasted & stunted
Acute malnutrition (Wasting)	**W/H Z score** (WHZ)	**W/H % of median** (WHM)	**MUAC** (cm) (6–59 mo)
Mild acute	$-2 \le z < -1$	80% ≤ % WHM < 90%	12.5 ≤ MUAC <13.5
Moderate acute (MAM)	$-3 \le z < -2$	70% ≤ % WHM < 80%	11.5 ≤ MUAC <12.5
Severe acute (SAM)	$z < -3$ or symmetrical edema	WHM < 70% or symmetrical edema	MUAC <11.5 or symmetrical edema
Global acute (GAM)	$z < -2$ or symmetrical edema	WHM < 80% or symmetrical edema	MUAC <12.5 or symmetrical edema
Underweight	**W/Age Z score** (WAZ)	**W/Age % of median** (WAM)	
Mild	$-2 \le z < -1$		
Moderate	$-3 \le z < -2$		
Severe	$z < -3$ or symmetrical edema		
Chronic malnutrition (Stunting)	**H/Age Z score** (HAZ)	**H/Age % of median** (HAM)	
Mild stunting	$-2 \le z < -1$		
Moderately stunted	$-3 \le z < -2$	85% ≤ HAM <90%	
Severely stunted	$z < -3$ or symmetrical edema	HAM <85% or symmetrical edema	

Note: in U2, length is the preferred term over height

Wasting

- WHO defines 3 types of severe malnutrition: severe wasting (SAM), severe stunting, and edematous malnutrition. This last includes kwashiorkor and marasmatic kwashiorkor in the Wellcome classification.
- SAM = severe wasting cases or bilateral pitting edema cases (where due to malnutrition)
- SAM = WHZ < −3, MUAC <11.5 cm, or bilateral pitting edema (WHO). WHM not in definition.
- SAM prevalence worldwide ≈ 20,000,000.
- SAM mortality ≈ 9x mortality of normally nourished child and its CFR can be 10–50%.
- GAM = MAM + SAM
- GAM = moderate wasting cases, severe wasting cases, or bilateral pitting edema cases (where due to malnutrition)

Underweight

- Underweight is not used for screening or surveys in nutritional emergencies. It reflects past (chronic) and present (acute) undernutrition and is unable to distinguish between them. It encompasses children who are wasted and/or stunted. However, weight gain over time can be a sensitive indicator of growth faltering which is easily tracked on Road to Health charts.

Stunting

- Stunting generally occurs before age 2. It is irreversible.
- Stunting prevalence worldwide ≈ 165,000,000.
- Stunting is not a good predictor of mortality, but the CFR from IDs in cases of severe stunting ≈ 3x the CFR from IDs in cases without stunting.

Reference standards can be absolute MUAC, centile, % of median reference, or z scores:

- MUAC
  Easy to understand. An excellent predictor of mortality. Permits comparisons between age groups insofar as the low growth velocity of MUAC in the U5 age group makes data roughly comparable. May be used alone in "quick-and-dirty" convenience samples to estimate local prevalence of wasting. However, not used alone in authoritative anthropometric surveys, and is commonly part of a two stage screening process to determine eligibility for feeding programs.
- Centiles
  Easy to understand. Permits comparisons between age groups and outliers. However, data are not convenient to convert.
  Eg z − 4.0 = 0.0032nd percentile
- % of Median of reference population
  WHM is the preferred indicator to determine eligibility for feeding programs (Sphere). Calculations are easy and are used in the WHO Road to Health Charts.
  However, median reference data are not comparable between ages.
  eg 60% wt-for-age = severe malnutrition in infants
  = moderate malnutrition in school age kids

Moreover, median reference data are not comparable between indicators.
eg 60% wt-for-age = severe malnutrition in infants
60% wt-for-ht = death

- Z scores
Preferred indicator (Sphere, WHO) for reporting anthropometry survey results because it permits comparisons between age groups and nutritional indices.
However, data may be difficult to understand.
eg z score wt-for-age for 1 y/o:

$$= \frac{wt_{Pt} - wt_{ref\ pop}}{SD_{ref\ pop}}$$

$$= \frac{6.1\ kg - 10.1\ kg}{1.0}$$

= – 4 SD below median for his age

Overall

WHZ gives higher prevalence of malnutrition than WHM for the same population. This is most marked where there is low baseline prevalence of disease, and especially for adolescents (who get subsequently over-referred).
WHZ is more statistically valid, but WHM is better predictor of mortality and is used for admission to TFCs.
Weight-for-age is influenced by weight-for-height and height-for-age. It can be difficult to interpret.

b. adults and adolescents (O10)
anthropometrics: BMI = weight (kg) / height $(m)^2$

Table 7.3.9
Anthropometric Indicators in Adults

Nutritional status	BMI (adults & adolescents)	MUAC (cm) (adults)	MUAC (cm) (pregnant & lactating)
Obese	30+		
Overweight	25 ≤ BMI < 30		
NL	18.5 ≤ BMI < 25		
Mild malnutrition	17 ≤ BMI < 18.5		
Moderate malnutrition	16 ≤ BMI < 17	16.0 ≤ MUAC <18.5	17.0 ≤ MUAC <18.5
Severe malnutrition	BMI < 16 or edema or < 5% of 10–18 yr reference population	MUAC <16.0 or edema	MUAC <17.0 or edema
Global (mod + severe)	BMI < 17 or edema	MUAC <18.5 or edema	MUAC <18.5 or edema

3. Population prevalence (U5)
   a. survey key attributes
      (1) representative at unit of analysis
      (2) robust (> 25 clusters recommended)
      (3) standardized (standardization test done)
      (4) data normally distributed (check standard deviation)
      (5) findings plausible (plausibility score)
   b. preferences for indicator and methods (IPC)
      (1) GAM by WHZ from representative survey >
      (2) GAM by WHZ from sentinel sites >
      (3) GAM by MUAC from representative survey >
      (4) GAM by MUAC from exhaustive screening >
      (5) GAM by MUAC from sentinel sites >
      (6) GAM by MUAC from screening

Malnutrition Classification

Table 7.3.10
Malnutrition Classification by Prevalence Range (WHO [5])

Malnutrition	Prevalence (%)			
	Acceptable (Low)	Poor (Med)	Serious (High)	Critical (Very high)
Wasting (GAM)	< 5	5–9	10–14	≥ 15
Underweight	< 10	10–19	20–29	≥ 30
Stunting	< 20	20–29	30–39	≥ 40

Source: World Health Organization. In: *Global Database on Child Growth and Malnutrition* © 2017. Used with permission of WHO.

Table 7.3.11
Malnutrition Classification by Prevalence Range (adapted from IPC [6])

Indicator	Prevalence (%)				
	Phase 1 Acceptable	Phase 2 Alert	Phase 3 Serious	Phase 4 Critical	Phase 5 Ext critical
GAM by WHZ % < −2 or edema	< 5	5–9.9	10–14.9	15–29.9	≥ 30
GAM by MUAC % < 12.5 cm or edema	< 6	6–10.9		11–16.9	≥ 17

Source: IPC Global Partners © 2016. Used with permission of IPC Global Partnership

Acute Food Security Classification

Table 7.3.12
Acute Food Security Reference Table (IPC [7])

Phase classification	**Reference data** (not all indicators required to determine classification)
Phase 1—Minimal Generally food secure (green)	CDR < 0.5/10,000/d, U5DR ≤ 1/10,000/d GAM < 5% Food consumption usually adequate (> 2100 kcal/p/d) Livelihood assets sustainable utilization
Phase 2—Stressed Borderline food insecure (yellow)	CDR < 0.5/10,000/d, U5DR ≤ 1/10,000/d GAM 5–10% Food consumption borderline adequate (2100 kcal/p/d) 20% + of HH c livelihood assets stressed & unsustainable utilization (livelihood deficit) Non-food expenditures (schools, health care) decrease
Phase 3—Crisis Acute food and livelihood crisis (orange)	CDR 0.5–1/10,000/d, U5DR 1–2/10,000/d GAM 10–15% or greater than usual and increasing 20% + of HH c food consumption gaps (< 2100 kcal/p/d or 2100 kcal/p/d via asset stripping) (survival deficit) Livelihood assets accelerated & critical depletion
Phase 4—Emergency (red)	CDR 1–2/10,000/d, U5DR > 2–4/10,000/d (excess mortality) GAM > 15–30% or greater than usual and increasing 20% + of HH c food consumption gaps marked (< 2100 kcal/p/d) Livelihood assets near complete & irreversible depletion
Phase 5—Famine (maroon)	CDR > 2/10,000/d, U5DR > 4/10,000/d GAM > 30% 20% + of HH c food consumption grossly inadequate (<< 2100 kcal/p/d) Livelihood assets complete loss

Source: IPC Global Partners © 2012. Used with permission of FAO-UN on behalf of IPC Global Partnership

4. Therapy

IPC Phase 2 needs livelihood support.
IPC Phase 3+ needs above plus nutritional support.

Table 7.3.13
Nutritional Support of Malnourished Population

Nutritional status	Therapy
Mild acute	Adequate general ration
Moderate acute (GAM > 10%)	Above + supplementary feeding or community therapeutic care (U5 + PLW)
Severe acute (SAM > 2%)	Therapeutic feeding, community therapeutic care, or hospitalization

General Food Distribution (GFD)

2100 kcal/p/d requires 12 kg food/p/mo or ≈ 15 kg food/p/mo in logistics pipeline.

Ration—WFP commonly aims for 50% ration in settings where resources are limited.

Cost—$1000/MT Title II bulk food from US sources

Preventive Intervention (for populations on edge of frank malnutrition)

Targeted—see SFP below

Community Management of Acute Malnutrition (CMAM)

4 Components:

<u>Stabilization Center (SC)</u>

- admission criteria: age 6–59 mo, SAM (MUAC <11.5 cm, WHZ < −3, or edema), anorexia, or severe medical complications
- treatment: F75, F100, IVF, ABX
- discharge criteria: appetite recovered, medical complication improved, pitting edema decreased, and clinically well

<u>Outpatient Therapeutic Program (OTP)</u>

- admission criteria: age 6–59 mo, SAM (MUAC <11.5 cm), appetite intact, and no severe medical complications
- treatment: RUTF (eg Plumpy'Nut® nutritionally = F100)
- discharge criteria: 15% weight gain (from entry weight), no bilateral pitting edema x 2 wks, and 2 mo minimum observation/treatment period

<u>Supplementary Feeding Program (SFP)</u>

- blanket—all HH in geographically targeted catchment area (eg where IPC 3+ and GAM > 15% or 10–14% with aggravating factors)
- targeted—some HH in catchment area (eg where GAM 10–14% or 5–9% with aggravating factors); U5 and pregnant or lactating women vs U5 alone vs U2 alone depending on resources available and challenges with case finding)

overall programmatic target—50% coverage for SAM in rural areas (Sphere); 30% coverage for MAM in rural areas
admission criteria
pedes: age 6–59 mo, MUAC <12.5 cm, with appetite, discharged from OTP, no severe medical complications
pregnant & lactating: MUAC <21.0 cm, and 2nd - 3rd trimester or with infant <6 mo
treatment: RUSF as dry rations eg Plumpy'Sup®, CSB, CSB + (supercereal), CSB ++ (supercereal +)
NB CSB may also be cooked on-site in emergency school feedings.
discharge criteria (pedes): weight gain, MUAC >12.5 cm, time in program >2 months

Community Outreach with Mobile Brigades

Therapeutic Feeding Program

Admission criteria for U5: SAM (WHZ < −3, MUAC <11.5 cm, or bilateral pitting edema)
Discharge criteria for U5: WHZ > −2.5, no edema, and clinically well (generally takes 4–6 weeks)
Treatment protocol (WHO, ICDDR)
Shock Severe dehydration: RL + D5, ½ strength Darrow's + D5, or ½ NS + D5
Dose: 100 cc/kg IV

Table 7.3.14
IV Therapy of Severe Dehydration

Age	Initial bolus	Balance
< 1 year	30 cc/kg IV over 1 h	70 cc/kg IV over 5 h
> 1 year	30 cc/kg IV over ½ h	70 cc/kg IV over 2 ½ h
If severely malnourished (WHO)	15 cc/kg IV over 1 h + ReSoMal 10 cc/kg by NGT	If improved after initial bolus, repeat 15 cc/kg IV over 1 h + ReSoMal 10 cc/kg/h PO/NGT x 10 h; If not improved after initial bolus, assume septic shock
If severely malnourished (ICDDR)	20 cc/kg IV over 1 h	10 cc/kg/h over 10 h + ORS 5–10 cc/kg PO after each loose stool

Dehydration

Moderate dehydration (5–10%): ReSoMal PO or NGT

With malnutrition: Dose 75–100 cc/kg PO/NGT over 12 h given as 5 cc/kg/half h × 4, then 5–10 cc/kg/h × 10 h (WHO)

Without malnutrition: Dose 75–100 cc/kg PO over 4 h (if age > 1 yr) or over 6 h (if < age 1 yr) (ICDDR)

NB ICDDR does not use ReSoMal but prefers rice-based ORS for all patients with diarrhea

Feeding c therapeutic milks—F75 (Phase 1), F100 (Phase 2)

D10 or F75 for hypoglycemia; blankets/warmer for hypothermia

3 Rx—ABX, mebendazole, antimalarial

Adjuncts—vitamins A-D, minerals, measles vaccine, Fe (only in rehab phase)

a. process indicators
   (1) daily average weight gain at TFC: > 8 g/kg/p
b. outcome indicators
   (1) cure
   (2) complications (~25% SAM will have medical complications)
   (3) death (~25% SAM will die with good care, and 50% will die with mediocre care)

Table 7.3.15
Exit Indicators in Therapeutic Feeding Programs

Setting /reference		Exit indicator			
		Cure	Mortality	Default	Non-response
TFC	Target (SPHERE)	> 75%	< 10%	< 15%	
	Target (NGO)	> 80%	< 5%	< 10%	
	Alert (NGO)	< 50%	> 15%	> 25%	
SFC	Target (SPHERE)	> 75%	< 3%	< 15%	
	Target (NGO)	> 75%	< 3%	< 15%	< 20%
	Alert (NGO)	< 50%	> 10%	> 30%	> 30%

C. Micronutrient Deficiency

Table 7.3.16
Micronutrient deficiency states

Micronutrients	Disease	Clinical findings
Vitamins		
A	Avitamnosis A	Night blindness, xerophthalmia, Bitot's spots, corneal ulcer/ keratomalacia, corneal scars
B_1 (Thiamine)	Beri-beri	Wet (acute)—congestive heart failure, anasarca; dry (chronic)—peripheral neuropathy (eg sensory Δs, wrist drop), weakness, weight loss, progressive ascending weakness (can't stand from a squat)
B_2 (Riboflavin)		Cheilosis, angular stomatitis, glossitis
B_3 (Niacin)	Pellagra	Dermatitis (sun-exposed areas eg Casal's necklace; tongue bright red), diarrhea, dementia, death
B_9 (Folate)	Anemia	Glossitis, others as per anemia below
C	Scurvy	Gingivitis, dental loosening, petechiae, delayed wound healing
D	Rickets	Bone-cartilage junctions enlarged at ribs (rachitic beads), wrists, & ankles; frontal bossing; sternal prominence; long bones bowed; joints with "splaying, cupping, & fraying"
Minerals		
I	Hypothyroid	Goiter, cretinism (mental retardation, short stature, squint, deaf-mutism)
Zn	Zinc deficiency	Diarrhea, delayed wound healing
Other Cofactors		
Fe	Anemia	Fatigue, dyspnea, pallor, mental dullness (#1 nutritional disorder in the world)

VIII. CHEMICAL WEAPONS

A. Chemical Agents

Table 7.3.17
Chemical Agent Characteristics, Clinical Effects, and Treatments

Chemical agents					
Agent	**Physical characteristics**	**Systems affected**	**Sx**	**Decon first aid**	**Tx antidote**
Blister Mustard (H, HD, HN)	Oily light yellow-brown liquids with odor of garlic	Eye—few hrs; resp & derm—2-24 hrs; **lethal in large doses**	Red skin, blisters, eye burning, coughing	Remove agent, S&W, flush with dilute bleach	None, supportive care
Blister Lewisite (L)	Oily colorless liquid with odor of geraniums	Derm—immediate pain; **lethal in large doses**	Skin pain or irritation, eye burning, coughing	Remove agent, S&W, flush with dilute bleach	BAL, supportive care
Blister Phosgene oxime (CX)	Solid <95 ° F but vaporizes	Derm—immediate pain **lethal in large doses**	Skin pain, wheals, eye burning, coughing	Remove agent, S&W, flush with dilute bleach	None, supportive care
Blood Cyanide (AC)	Rapid evaporating liquids with odor of bitter almonds; gas lighter than air	Resp, heme—death in min; **highly lethal**	Cherry red skin or lips, rapid respirations, dizziness, HA, seizures, death	Usually none; leave area, aeration, S&W	Amyl nitrite, Na thiosulfate
Blood Cyanogen Cl (CK)	Rapid evaporating liquids with odor of bitter almonds; gas heavier than air	Resp, heme—death in min; **highly lethal**	Cherry red skin or lips, rapid respirations, dizziness, HA, seizures, death	Usually none; leave area, aeration, S&W	Amyl nitrite, Na thiosulfate
Choking Phosgene (CG)	Rapid evaporating liquid with odor of mown hay	Resp, derm—death in days; **lethal in large doses**	Eye and resp irritation	Leave area, aeration, S&W, eye irrigation	None, supportive care

Chemical agents					
Agent	**Physical characteristics**	**Systems affected**	**Sx**	**Decon first aid**	**Tx antidote**
Choking Chlorine (Cl)	Gas at room temp	Resp—death in days; **lethal in large doses**	Eye & resp irritation, chest tightness, delayed pulm edema	Leave area, aeration, S&W, eye irrigation	None, supportive care
Nerve Tabun (GA), Sarin (GB), Soman (GD)	Colorless, odorless liquid; G agents less volatile than water	Resp—seconds to minutes; derm—min to hrs; **highly lethal**	Blurry vision, twitching, chest tightness, SOB SLUDGE, brady,broncho-spasm, seizures	Remove agent, S&W, flush with dilute bleach	Atropine, 2-PAM
Nerve VX	Slight yellow colored liquid at room temp; V agents as volatile as motor oil	Resp—seconds to minutes; derm—min to hrs; **highly lethal**	Blurry vision, twitching, chest tightness, SOB SLUDGE, brady,broncho-spasm, seizures	Remove agent, S&W, flush with dilute bleach	Atropine, 2-PAM
Riot control Tear gas (CS), Mace (CN)	Gas at room temp	Resp—seconds; non-lethal	Eye & resp irritation	Leave area, aeration, S&W, eye irrigation	None

BAL British anti-Lewisite
2-PAM 2-pyridine aldoxime methyl chloride
S&W soap and water
SLUDGE salivation, lacrimation, urination, defecation, GI distress, emesis
SOB shortness of breath

B. Management of MCI from Suspected Chemical Weapons
(adapted from Domestic Preparedness Training [8])
Overarching rule: all responders should wear personal protective equipment to avoid becoming a victim.

Notification Phase (RAIN)

1. **R**ecognize a problem
   a. mass casualties
   b. syndromic casualty pattern
   c. dissemination device
   d. warning from perpetrator
   e. patient (host)—compelling symptoms
   f. agent—identifiable sights or smells
   g. environment—dead animals

2. **A**void
   a. distance—100 m from chemical attack, 300 m from explosion
   b. direction—upwind, upgrade, upstream
   c. 4 don'ts—don't become a victim, don't rush in, don't TEST (taste, eat, smell, touch), don't assume anything
3. **I**solate
   a. cordon off the area to extent possible
   b. isolate the casualties
4. **N**otify authorities
   a. informant
   b. agent released
   c. immediate M & M
   d. signs and symptoms
   e. type of device/vehicle/container—specify sights, smells, sounds
   f. secondary disaster of fire or explosion
   g. wind direction, weather conditions
   h. witnesses
   i. lead responder
   j. actions taken
   k. actions forthcoming
   l. meeting place for responders
   m. follow-up contact (time, means, channel)

Response Phase

1. Site security
   a. position equipment upwind, upgrade, and upstream from incident site
   b. isolate the area including downwind vapor hazard area
   c. establish hot (ambient hazard), warm (contaminated victims), and cold (clean treatment) zones
2. Staff protection
   a. PPE for providers in the hot zone
   b. ICS to manage the incident
   c. SOPs to guide responder actions
3. Social controls (PINS)
   a. **P**reserve evidence
   b. **I**dentify the agent
   c. **N**eutralize contaminated areas
   d. **S**earch for secondary devices
4. Environmental and case management
   a. corral casualties and victims
   b. establish decontamination stations
   c. perform decontamination
   d. provide first aid—triage, treat, transport

Emergency Self-decontamination

1. Wet or blot (blotting for chemical contamination; wetting down for bio or nuclear contamination)
2. Strip off clothing
3. Flush the affected area with water or dilute bleach
4. Cover the affected area

C. Implications for Disaster Management

1. Forensic
2. Clinical
3. Epidemiological
4. Pharmacological
5. Environmental
6. Social
7. Judicial
8. Political

IX. EPI METHODS

A. Rates

1. Death rates—calculated incidence of death expressed per 10,000 p/d or per 1000 p/mo; data collected by retrospective surveys (eg 3 month period) to gauge severity of public health emergency particularly where sudden events lead to spike in mortality
   a. CDR—crude death rate
   b. ASDR—age-specific death rate (eg U5DR or death rate of children 0–5 yr) during a studied time interval (written as $_5M_0$ or 0-5DR); age of study cohort, eg 0–5 yr, should not be confused with study time intervals

Table 7.3.18
Representative death rates

Situation	CDR	0-5DR
Baseline in developing countries	< < 1	1
Emergency under control	< 1	< 2
Serious trouble	1–2	2–4
Emergency out of control	> 2	> 4
Catastrophe	> 4	

2. Mortality rates—calculated probability of dying before a specified age expressed per 1000 live births; data collected by national health authorities in periodic (annual) demographic surveys to reflect ongoing health status
   a. CMR—calculated probability of mortality in given population for specific time

b. IMR—calculated probability of a live borne child dying before 1 yr

c. U5MR—calculated probability of a live borne child dying before 5 yr

NB MR ≠ DR. Eg CMR ≠ CDR, U5MR ≠ U5DR. Different rates measure different things and are not directly comparable. However, MRs may be converted into DRs by the following: CDR or U5DR (deaths/10,000/d) = – ln(1–p/1000) × 5.47 where p = CMR or U5MR (deaths/1000 live births). However, this has little field utility.

NB MMR—maternal mortality ratio has different units in numerators (maternal deaths) and denominators (live births), thus is a ratio, not a rate

B. Conclusions

Interpolation

The application of study findings to an entire population from which the sample was drawn. If the survey was well-conducted, the results may be considered representative of the entire population. This is scientifically justified. However a confidence interval should accompany any parameter estimate of that population.

Extrapolation

The extension of study findings to a population or period which was not represented in the sample. It works by association—if 2 populations appear to be experiencing similar conditions, the morbidity/mortality experience of one may be imputed to the other. This is not scientifically justified, but is often done where data are insufficient or impossible to collect.

References

1. Declaration of Alma-Ata. International Conference on Primary Health Care, Alma-Ata, USSR, 6–12 September 1978. Available from: http://www.who.int/publications/almaata_declaration_en.pdf?ua=1.
2. Walsh J, Warren K. Selective primary health care—an interim strategy for disease control in developing countries. *N Engl J Med* 1979; 301:967–74.
3. Mara D, Feachem RG. Water and excreta-related diseases: unitary environmental classification. *Journal of Environmental Engineering, April 1999*; 125(4):334–9.
4. Feachem RG. Infections related to water and excreta: the health dimension of the decade. In: *Water Supply and Sanitation in Developing Countries*. London: Institution of Water Engineers and Scientists, 1983.
5. World Health Organization. Global database on child growth and malnutrition. Available from: https://www.who.int/nutgrowthdb/about/introduction/en/index5.html. Accessed June 9, 2017.

6. IPC Global Partners. Addendum to IPC Technical Manual Version 2.0. Tools and procedures for classification of acute malnutrition. Rome: IPC Global Partnership, 2016. p 14.
7. IPC Global Partners. Integrated Food Security Phase Classification Technical Manual Version 2.0. Evidence and Standards for Better Food Security Decisions. Rome: FAO-UN on behalf of IPC Global Partners, 2012. p 32.
8. NBC Domestic Preparedness Training Hospital Provider Course. Undated. Curriculum available from: Center for Domestic Preparedness, Anniston AL, http://cdp.dhs.gov/.

Document 7.4
TROPICAL MEDICINE

Glossary

abd	abdomen
ABX	antibiotics
ACP	asymptomatic cyst passer
ACT	artemisinin-based combination therapy
AF	acid-fast (eg Ziehl-Neelsen)
AFP	acute flaccid paralysis
Ag	antigen
aggl	agglutination
AHF	acute hepatic failure
AIDS	acquired immunodeficiency syndrome
AR	attack rate
ARDS	acute respiratory distress syndrome
ARF	acute renal failure
ARI	acute respiratory infection
ART	antiretroviral therapy
Aus	Australia
AVB	atrioventricular block
BAL	bronchoalveolar lavage
BC	blood culture
BM	bone marrow
BW (A, B)	biological weapon, biological warfare (threat class)
Bx	biopsy
c	century; with
C	centigrade; chills
CA	Central America
Ca	cancer
CE	complex emergency
CFR	case fatality ratio
CHF	congestive heart failure
CI	chronic illnesses
CMI	cell-mediated immunity
CMP	cardiomyopathy
CNS	central nervous system
CP	complications
CSF	cerebrospinal fluid
CT	chemotherapy; cholera toxin; computed tomography
d	day(s)
D	diarrhea
DAA	direct-acting antivirals
DC	developing country
DDx	differential diagnosis
DF	dengue fever
DIC	disseminated intravascular coagulation
DOTS	directly observed therapy short course
DRC	Democratic Republic of the Congo

Dx	diagnosis
E	east, eastern
EAEC	enteroadherent *E. coli*
EHEC	enterohemorrhagic *E. coli*
EIEC	enteroinvasive *E. coli*
ELISA	enzyme-linked immunosorbent assay
EM	erythema migrans
ENL	erythema nodosum leprosum
ETEC	enterotoxigenic *E. coli*
Eur	Europe
exts	extremities
F	female; fever
FAR	fever, arthritis, and rash
FO	fecal-oral
FQ	fluoroquinolone
FSU	former Soviet Union
FTT	failure to thrive
FUO	fever of unknown origin
GB	gall bladder
GBS	Guillain-Barre syndrome
GI	gastrointestinal
GIB	gastrointestinal bleed
H2H	human-to-human (transmission)
HA	headache
HAV	hepatitis A virus
HB	heart block; hepatitis B
HBIG	hepatitis B immunoglobulin
HBV	hepatitis B virus
HCC	hepatocellular carcinoma
HD	heart disease
HeAn	hemolytic anemia
hemor	hemorrhage
HF	hemorrhagic fever
HIV	human immunodeficiency virus
HM	hepatomegaly
HSM	hepatosplenomegaly
HSV	herpes simplex virus
HTN	hypertension
HUS	hemolytic-uremic syndrome
HZ	herpes zoster
I	incidence
IC	industrialized country
ICP	immunocompromised person
ID	infectious disease
ID_{50}	median infectious dose
IDU	injecting drug user
IE	infective endocarditis
IFA	immunofluorescence assay
IG	immune (serum) globulin
JH	Jarisch-Herxheimer (reaction)
LA	Latin America (Central America + South America)
LBRF	louse-borne relapsing fever
LBTF	louse-borne typhus fever
LBW	low birth weight

LE	lower extremity
LF	Lassa fever
LGV	lymphogranuloma venereum
LN	lymph node, lymphadenopathy
Lx	laboratory
M	male
MB	multibacillary
MDR	multidrug resistant
ME	Middle East
MM	mucous membranes
MODS	multiple organ dysfunction syndrome
MS	mental status
N	nausea; north, northern
NA	North America
NAf	North Africa
NFI	nerve function impairment
NH	northern hemisphere
NL	normal
NV	nausea and vomiting
OD	opportunistic disease
OI	opportunistic infection
org	pathological organism
p	after
P	prevalence
PB	paucibacillary
PCN	penicillin
PCR	polymerase chain reaction
PEP	post-exposure prophylaxis
perf	perforation
PGL	persistent generalized lymphadenopathy
PMN	polymorphonuclear leukocyte
PNG	Papua New Guinea
PS	peripheral blood smear
Pt	patient
PUD	peptic ulcer disease
Px	physical exam
RBBB	right bundle branch block
RDT	rapid diagnostic test
RHZE	rifampicin + isoniazid + pyrazinamide + ethambutol
RTPCR	reverse transcriptase polymerase chain reaction
RUQ	right upper quadrant
Rx	drug therapy
s	without
S	south, southern
SA	South America
SAFE	surgery, antibiotics, facial cleanliness, environmental improvement
SAM	severe acute malnutrition
SBE	subacute bacterial endocarditis
SC	stool culture
SD1	*S. dysenteriae* type 1
SE	southeast
SM	splenomegaly
SSA	sub-Saharan Africa

SSD	sickle cell disease	UE	upper extremity
s/sx	signs and symptoms	US	ultrasound
STEC	shiga toxin-producing *E. coli*	UTI	urinary tract infection
STI	sexually transmitted infection	V	vomiting
sx	symptoms	VBD	vector-borne disease
sz	seizure	VE	viral encephalitis
TB	tuberculosis	VHF	viral hemorrhagic fever
TIG	tetanus immune globulin	VL	visceral leishmaniasis
TMP/SMZ	trimethoprim + sulfamethoxazole	W	west, western
TPE	tropical pulmonary eosinophilia	wk	week
Tx	treatment	YF	yellow fever
U5	under 5 year-old	Δ	change in
UC	urine culture	//	similar to

Pathophysiology

Why does this person from this place get this disease at this time?

Person Think of new exposure for Pts from non-endemic or developed areas. Think of breakdown in immunity for Pts from endemic or undeveloped areas.

For systemic infection, infective dose is a function of immunity and innoculum.

immunity relates to host and may be altered by congenital, acquired, or iatrogenic causes

innoculum relates to infectious organism and the environment

Place Think geographic medicine.

Time Think seasonality. Malaria is classic:

- Holo-endemic areas (eg Congo) have an intense level of malaria transmission year-round. Epidemics don't occur unless displacement brings in non-immune populations. Infection may be asymptomatic. Effective partial immunity develops in adults which enables clinical tolerance of infection and protects against serious episodes. Mortality is highest in pedes U5 and pregnant women.
- Hyper-endemic areas (eg W. Africa) have an intense but unstable level of transmission in seasonal peaks when the climatic conditions are favorable. Epidemics occur. Infection is generally symptomatic. Partial immunity fails to develop. Mortality occurs across all age groups.
- Hypo-endemic areas (eg Thai-Burmese border) have a low level of transmission year-round. Epidemics occur. Infection is generally symptomatic. Partial immunity fails to develop. Mortality occurs across all age groups.

S/Sx Think differential diagnosis (below).

Differential Diagnosis or Special Considerations in Common Presentations

Diarrhea

watery (secretory, small intestine)

viruses; *E. coli* (ETEC, EAEC), campylobacter, salmonella, vibrio, bacillus, *C. perfringens*; enteric protozoa except entamoeba

NB giardia, cryptosporidium often yield frothy D due to gut malabsorption

bloody (inflammatory, large intestine)

E. coli (EHEC or STEC eg O157:H7, EIEC), campylobacter, salmonella, shigella, *C. difficile*, yersinia; entamoeba

Dyspnea hantavirus pulmonary syndrome and pneumonic plague present similarly and are co-endemic

Fever < 7 d

PMNs > focal bacterial infections + lepto, amoeba (liver abscess), borrelia, sepsis (non-typhi salmonella, pneumococcus, staph, strep, meningococcus)

PMNs < or NL	rickettsia, malaria, typhoid, viruses
s localizing signs	sepsis (non-typhi salmonella, pneumococci, staph, strep, meningococcus), malaria, UTI, typhoid, HIV Lx: malaria smear, BC, UC, serology
rash/hemorrhage	as for fever s focal bacterial infections or amoeba
petechial rash	meningococcal sepsis, IE, DIC, Henoch-Schonlein purpura, VHF
jaundice	bacteria/parasite (coxiella, lepto, malaria, sepsis); SSD; viruses (YF, hepatitis); worms (ascaris, echinococcus, liver flukes)

Fever > 7 d

PMNs >	leprosy (erythema nodosum leprosum), amoeba (liver abscess), borrelia, deep sepsis
Eos >	tissue nematodes, zoonotic nematodes, strongyloides > other gut nematodes c heart-lung migration, cestodes (excluding gut tapeworms), trematodes
PMNs NL	brucella, chronic meningococcal sepsis, SBE, syphilis, TB (localized), toxo, tryps
PMNs <	brucella, HIV, malaria, TB (disseminated), typhoid, VL

NB fever + Δ ABCD = emergency
fever + any 2 = potentially lethal lesion (eg fever + jaundice + acute renal failure)
afebrile failure to thrive in infants is worked up like fever without localizing signs
borrelia // lepto in acute fevers; coxiella // brucella in chronic fevers

Hepatomegaly hepatitis, hepatoma, hepatic abscess, hydatid, schisto, TB, malaria

Jaundice

prehepatic	malaria, sepsis, hemolysis, hemoglobinopathy
hepatic	viral hepatitis, YF, Q fever, lepto, drugs
post-hepatic	gallstones, choledochocarcinoma, hydatid in biliary tree, ascariasis in biliary tree, liver flukes

Neuro signs unexplained TB, HIV and OIs, syphilis, Lyme disease, Whipple's disease, brain abscess

Paralysis

flaccid	Guillain-Barre syndrome (immune mediated), polio (anterior horn infection)
spastic	trauma, vascular, neoplasm, infection—HIV/HTLV, abscess, TB, subacute combined degeneration

Splenomegaly—massive

congestive	SSD, schisto
reactive	malaria
infiltrative	amyloid, VL, lymphoma, leukemia
combined	

Splenomegaly—moderate

above + differential diagnosis for F > 7 d c PMNs < or NL

STI—bubo

ulcer	chancroid, granuloma inguinale
no ulcer	LGV
no STD	plague, filariasis, LE infection

STI—ulcer

single, painless	1° syphilis (s LN), LGV (transient, c bubo), granuloma inguinale (progressive c pseudobuboes) granuloma diseases start with one painless ulcer, but develop painful bubos
single, painful	superinfection of painless lesion, TB
mult, painless	2° syphilis
mult, painful	herpes (often c systemic Sx & LN), chancroid (c bubo)

BW syndromes

influenza	many BW agents initially present as flu-like syndrome (F, C, HA, malaise, myalgia)
pulmonary	anthrax*, plague, tularemia, Q fever, melioidosis, hantavirus
jaundice	HA
encephalitis	VE, Q fever
rash, cutaneous	smallpox*, tularemia, typhus fever
septicemia/shock	anthrax*, plague, typhus fever, VHF
occult death	

* not further characterized as tropical disease in Tables 7.4.1 & 7.4.2 below

Vectors and Intermediate Hosts

Vector—comes to you (not necessarily required for development of the organism)
mosquitoes and ticks transmit the most types of infectious pathogens
Aedes transmit all mosquito-vectored VHF

Intermediate hosts—you come to the intermediate host (required for development of the organism)
intestinal nematodes have none
all trematodes +1 zoonotic nematode require snails

Management Keys

Keep a broad differential diagnosis in mind: trauma, vessel, neoplasia, infection, drugs, toxins, congenital, metabolic, endocrine, nutrition, connective tissue diseases (autoimmune), psyc

Know the local epidemiology.
Leading U5 causes of death worldwide—LRI (15%), prematurity (15%), birth asphyxia (11%), diarrhea (9%), malaria (7%), neonatal sepsis (7%)
Leading ID causes of death worldwide—LRI, diarrhea, HIV/AIDS, TB, malaria, measles, meningitis

Know the golden rules of infectious diseases.

Golden Rules of Infectious Diseases (abstracted from A Yung [1] and used with permission)

1. Rigors are always important—serious bacterial infections are the most likely cause.
2. Severe muscle pain may be a symptom of sepsis even without fever.
3. Elderly patients with sepsis may be afebrile. In elderly patients, fever is rarely caused by a viral infection.
4. Septic patients who are hypothermic have a worse prognosis than those with high fever. Treat as a medical emergency.
5. Fever in a postoperative patient is usually related to the surgical procedure (eg pneumonia, UTI, wound, or deep infection).
6. Fever with jaundice is rarely due to viral hepatitis. Think liver abscess, cholangitis, etc.
7. The rash of early meningococcal infection may resemble a viral rash.
8. Generalized rashes involving the palms and soles may be due to drugs, viral infections, rickettsial infections, or syphilis.
9. All febrile travelers in or returned from a malaria infected area must have malaria excluded.
10. Disseminated TB must be suspected in all elderly patients with fever and multisystem disease who have been in an area with endemic TB.
11. Septic arthritis may be present even in a joint which is mobile.
12. Back pain with fever may be caused by vertebral osteomyelitis or an epidural abscess.
13. A patient may have more than one infection requiring treatment (eg malaria and typhoid), especially if they are elderly, immunosuppressed, or have travelled.
14. Always remember common infections, not just opportunistic infections, in AIDS patients with a fever.

Understand morbidity multipliers—measles, malnutrition, and TB/HIV.

Understand occult co-morbidities.

For any undifferentiated illness, even in infants, think of HIV, TB, syphilis, and sarcoid.

For any child, think of malaria, hookworm, and anemia. Malarial anemia usually in pedes <3 year-old; hookworm anemia usually in pedes >3 year-old.

For any ICP, think of TB, VL, histoplasmosis, and strongyloides. Must treat early.

Watch for clinical mimics—malaria presenting as pneumonia or diarrhea in pedes; VL presenting as malaria in adults; lepto presenting as mild DF (esp in DF endemic areas where the Pt has mild onset of illness, worsening course, and no rash but jaundice).

Tx Do basic things well, use equipment you understand, teach others, delegate.

Table 7.4.1a
Tropical Infectious Diseases – Vector-Borne and Zoonotic

Vectors [Reservoir]	Organism	Arboviral and Zoonotic Viral Diseases						Annual Incidence or Prevalence	Deaths/year or CFR Rx, Vaccine
		Group/name	Clinical				Misc		
			FAR	CNS	VHF	H2H			
		Fever, Arthritis, & Rash (FAR)	Acute Sx over 2–6 d – F, C, HA, back pain, arthralgia, mac-pap rash, desquamation; recovery over 2–3 wks				Incubation <3 wk Lx – serology, ELISA, PCR H2H – Zika		
Mosquitoes (F)									
Aedes	Alphavirus	Chikungunya Virus Disease (Kimakonde verb – to be contorted)	+				Epidemic poly-arthritis (favors wrists, hands, ankles, feet)	SSA, S & SE Asia, Caribbean	Very rare no vaccine
Anopheles [humans]	Alphavirus	O'nyong-nyong	+				Epidemic poly-arthritis	SSA	0
Aedes, Culex	Alphavirus	Ross River Fever	+				Epidemic poly-arthritis	Australia	0
Culex	Alphavirus	Sindbis Virus Disease (Ockelbo disease, Pogosta disease)	+				Flu-like illness over 5d; CP of persisting arthritis	I-100 s foci worldwide not NA, LA	0

Aedes aegypti, albopictus [humans—urban; monkeys—rural]	Flavivirus (4 serotypes) **BW (A)**	Dengue Fever (DF) (breakbone fever)	+	+			Severe disease c F, C, retroorbital HA, back pain, myalgia, arthralgia, morbilliform rash; CP of DHF	I-100,000,000 apparent 300,000,000 inapparent #1 viral VBD Asia, LA, SSA; rainy season	< 1% vaccine in trial
Culex	Flavivirus **BW (B)**	West Nile Fever (WNF)	+	+			Mild disease c F, malaise, HA, myalgia, anorexia, NV, rash → CNS (1%)	Africa, ME, Eur, NA, CA; early fall in NH	c CNS, 25% c FAR, 0% no vaccine
Aedes	Flavivirus	Zika Fever (from Zika Forest in Uganda)	+			+ (STI)	Generally mild disease c F, malaise, HA, arthralgia, rash; neonatal microcephaly if contracted early in utero	Africa, Asia, Polynesia, SA	<< 1% from GBS and birth defects no vaccine
Sandflies (F)									
Phlebotomus	Bunyavirus	Sandfly Fever (phlebotomus fever, 3 day fever, pappataci fever)	+					S Europe, N Africa, E Mediterranean to N India	Very rare

(continued)

Table 7.4.1a (continued)

Vectors [Reservoir]	Organism	Arboviral and Zoonotic Viral Diseases						Annual Incidence or Prevalence	Deaths/year or CFR Rx, Vaccine
		Group/name	Clinical				Misc		
Phlebotomus	Rhabdovirus	Vesicular Stomatitis Virus (vesicular stomatitis fever)	+	+					Very rare
Ticks (M & F)									
Dermacentor (wood tick)	Reovirus	Colorado Tick Fever (CTF) (mountain tick fever)	+	+	+		Biphasic illness over 6 d; rare CP of Δ CNS, VHF	W NA; summer	Very rare no vaccine
		Viral Encephalitis (VE)	Most infections asymptomatic; severe infections c F, HA, Δ MS, meningeal signs				Incubation <3 wk Lx—serology, ELISA, PCR H2H—Nipah		
Mosquitoes (F)									
Culiseta, Aedes [birds]	Alphavirus **BW (B)**	Eastern Equine E (EEE)		+			Often severe	Rare E NA, CA, SA	25–50% esp pedes vaccine for horses, but not humans

Culex, Culiseta [birds]	Alphavirus **BW (B)**	Western Equine E (WEE)		+			Milder than EEE	Rare W NA, CA, SA	5% vaccine for horses, but not humans
Aedes, Culex, et al [rodents, birds, horses]	Alphavirus **BW (B)**	Venezuelan Equine E (VEE)	+	+				Large epidemics SA (esp Venezuela), CA, NA	< 1% vaccine for horses, but not humans
Aedes [squirrels, lagomorphs]	Bunyavirus (serogroup c La Crosse E) **BW (B)**	California E		+				I-100 esp pedes W NA; summer, fall	< 1% no vaccine
Culex [water fowl, pigs]	Flavivirus **BW (B)**	Japanese E (JE)		+			99 + % s Sx; 50% of survivors c neuro disability	I-70,000 esp pedes E Asia, S Asia, W Pacific	10,000 esp U5 20–30% vaccine
Culex [water fowl]	Flavivirus	Murray Valley E (MVE) (Australian E)		+			99% + s Sx; 40% of survivors c neuro disability	Australia, PNG; summer monsoon season	25% no vaccine
Culex [birds]	Flavivirus **BW (B)**	St. Louis E (SLE)		+				NA, CA; summer, fall	5–15% no vaccine

(continued)

Table 7.4.1a (continued)

Vectors [Reservoir]	Organism	Arboviral and Zoonotic Viral Diseases						Annual Incidence or Prevalence	Deaths/year or CFR Rx, Vaccine
		Group/name	Clinical				Misc		
Ticks (M & F)									
Ixodes [wild rodents]	Flavivirus (3 subtypes— European, Siberian, Far-eastern)	Tick-borne E (TBE)		+			Biphasic illness—febrile phase c flu-like Sx → neuro phase c Δ CNS	I-5000 Eur, FSU, Asia; summer, fall esp rural & recreational areas	1–2% vaccine
[Mammals]									
Horses, fruit bats	Hendra Virus	Hendra Virus Disease		+			Pneumonia early	Australia	50% vaccine for horses, but not humans
Pigs, fruit bats via urine or saliva contaminated fruits	Nipah Virus	Nipah Virus Disease		+		+	Flu-like Sx initially	S Asia	50% vaccine for primates, but not humans

Dogs, foxes, coyotes, skunks, raccoons, bats (infectious saliva)	Rabies Virus	Rabies (hydrophobia)	F, HA → 2 syndromes: encephalitic (furious) rabies (80%)—intermittent agitation & terror // mania alt c lucid intervals, autonomic hyper-activity, bulbar spasm to water (hydrophobia), spasticity, sz → **death in days**; paralytic rabies (20%)—ascending sensorimotor AFP, fasciculation, paraparesis, bulbar paralysis s hydrophobia → **death in wks**				Serology; skin Bx for IFA	Worldwide mostly in developing countries; 50% of people bitten by infected animal contract disease	50,000 s Tx 100% vaccine
		Viral Hemorrhagic Fever (VHF)	F, malaise, HA, conjunctivitis, pharyngitis, myalgia, arthralgia, rash (morbilliform to petechial); CP of Δ vasc perm, bleeding, shock, ARF, AHF, MODS				Incubation <3 wk Lx—serology, ELISA, PCR H2H—many but only from Pt c Sx		
Mosquitoes (F)									
Aedes, Culex, et al [livestock via inoculation or inhalation; abortion storm heralds human transmission risk]	Bunyavirus **BW (A)**	Rift Valley Fever (RVF)		+	+		5% c Δ CNS or HF	Sporadic epidemics NAf, SSA, ME	Overall <1% VHF 50% ribavirin; vaccine for animals, but not humans

(continued)

Table 7.4.1a (continued)

Vectors [Reservoir]	Organism	Arboviral and Zoonotic Viral Diseases						Annual Incidence or Prevalence	Deaths/year or CFR Rx, Vaccine
		Group/name	Clinical				Misc		
Aedes aegypti, albopictus [humans—urban; monkeys—rural]	Flavivirus (4 serotypes)	Dengue HF/ Dengue Shock Syndrome (DHF/ DSS)		+	+		Biphasic illness— F phase then cap leak c 4 clinical classes	I-500,000 pedes <15 S, SE Asia, W Pacific; rainy season	25,000 s Tx > 20% c Tx 2% no vaccine
Aedes aegypti, et al [humans—urban; monkeys—rural]	Flavivirus	Yellow Fever (YF)			+		F, C, HA, NV, jaundice; CP (20%) of AHF, GIB, ARF	I-200,000 endemic SSA (90% cases) > sporadic LA not Asia	30,000 endemic 10% sporadic 50% vaccine
Ticks (M & F)									
Hyalomma via tick bite or direct contact with blood from infected animal or human	Bunyavirus **BW (A)**	Congo-Crimea HF (CCHF)			+	+	Flu-like Sx—F, HA, eye pain, myalgias, abd pain, hepatitis; CP of hemor **rapidly fatal (2 wks) s Tx**	Central, S Asia, Africa; esp butchers, shepherds	20–50% ribavirin; no vaccine
Haemaphysalis [rodents, shrews]	Flavivirus	Kyasanur Forest Disease (monkey fever)		+	+		Flu-like Sx—F, HA, myalgias; CP of hemor in biphasic illness	I-500 India	3–5%

Dermacentor	Flavivirus	Omsk HF			+		Flu-like Sx—F, C, HA, myalgias, palatal rash, cervical LN; CP of hemor, Δ CNS	FSU esp Siberia	1–3%
[Mammals]									
Calomys (rodents) via aerosols from urine, saliva, or stool, or food con-tamination	Arenavirus **BW (A)**	Argentine HF (Junin)			+		VHF // LF, but 1/3 of untreated cases become severe c hemor and neuro signs	I-100 C Argentina; Mar-Apr; farm workers at corn harvest	s Tx 20% c Tx < 2% vaccine
Calomys (rodents) via aerosols from urine, saliva, or stool, or food con-tamination	Arenavirus **BW (A)**	Bolivian HF (Machupo) (black typhus)			+	+ (Low)	VHF Sx + low back pain	Bolivia	s Tx 20%
Rodents suspected via aerosols from urine, saliva, or stool, or food contamination	Arenavirus	Brazilian HF (Sabia)			+		VHF // LF, but 1/3 of untreated cases become severe c hemor and neuro signs	Brazil	no vaccine

(continued)

Table 7.4.1a (continued)

Vectors [Reservoir]	Organism	Arboviral and Zoonotic Viral Diseases						Annual Incidence or Prevalence	Deaths/year or CFR Rx, Vaccine
		Group/name	Clinical				Misc		
Sigmodon, et al (cotton rat, cane mouse) via aerosols from urine, saliva, or stool, or food contamination	Arenavirus **BW (A)**	Venezuelan HF (Guanarito)			+		VHF // LF, but 1/3 of untreated cases become severe c hemor and neuro signs	W Venezuela; Nov-Jan	s Tx > 30% no vaccine
Mastomys, et al (rodents) via aerosols or direct contact with stool or urine	Arenavirus **BW (A)**	Lassa Fever (LF)			+	+ (High)	Most s Sx; VHF Sx in 4 phases: F, malaise, fatigue (1–3 d); HA, sore throat, myalgia, DNV, cough (4–7 d); edema, bleeding (20% of Pt c Sx), Δ CNS (7+ d); coma (14 d); deafness common in survivors	100,000–300,000 W SSA; Jan-May; most common VHF c H2H in travelers	5000; 2–20% ribavirin; experimental vaccine
Mastomys (rodents)	Arenavirus **BW (A)**	Lujo HF			+	+	VHF Sx	< 10 in history S Africa, Zambia	s Tx 80%

Apodemus, et al (field mice) via bites or aerosols from urine, saliva, or stool	Bunyavirus (Hantavirus is 1 of 5 genera)	Hemorrhagic Fever with Renal Syndrome (HFRS) (Korean hemorrhagic fever from Hantan River area in S Korea)			+		5 phases: F, HA, malaise, back pain, NV, conj injection, rash (3–7 d); ↓ BP due to hemor (1–3 d); oliguria (3–7 d); diuresis (wks); recovery (months)	E Asia, Eur, NA, SA; late fall, early winter	c Tx 5–15% ribavirin; experimental vaccine
Peromyscus, et al (deer mice) as above	Bunyavirus (Hantavirus is 1 of 5 genera) **BW (A)**	Hantavirus Pulmonary Syndrome (hantavirus ARDS)				+ (Low)	Cardiopulmonary syndrome	As above; only Andes variant capable of H2H transmission	c Tx 30–40% no vaccine
? fruit bats → gorillas, duikers via saliva contamina-ted dropped fruits	Filovirus (5 types of Ebola; Sudan strain mildest) **BW (A)**	Ebola-Marburg Diseases (EHF, African HF)			+	+	VHF Sx + DNV; VHF CP (50% of Pt c hemor); **rapidly fatal s Tx**	SSA	Ebola 60–90% Marburg 30% experimental vaccine

Table 7.4.1b
Tropical Infectious Diseases—Vector-Borne and Zoonotic

Vectors [Reservoir]	Organism	Non-viral Diseases			Annual Incidence or Prevalence	Deaths/year or CFR Rx
		Name	Clinical	Lab Diagnosis		
Bugs (M & F)						
Triatoma (cone-nosed, kissing bugs) via direct contact with vector feces, food contamination, or congenital [humans in chronic disease]	*Trypano-soma cruzi*	American Trypanosomiasis (Chagas' disease)	Acute—chagoma, F, LN, HSM; chronic (25%)—HD (CMP, RBBB, CHF), megacolon	Amastigotes in tissue Bx; tryps in stained PS (rare); serology	I-300,000 P-10,000,000 LA (3rd most common VBD p malaria & DF)	11,000 rare acutely nifurtimox
Fleas (M & F)						
Xenopsylla via feces [rodents, feral cats, opossums]	*Rickettsia typhi*	Typhus Fever (FBTF) (endemic, murine)	// LBTF but milder	Serology	Worldwide; warm climates esp summer-fall	1–5% doxycycline

Xenopsylla, Pulex via regurgitation, direct contact c org from infected HH pets [rodents]	*Yersinia pestis* **BW (A)**	Plague	Bubonic—sudden onset F, C, extreme malaise, myalgia, tender LN at site of inoculation (<u>bubo</u>); CP of sepsis, pneumonia (pneumonic plague), meningitis, DIC; 10–25% of plague cases have primary septicemia; **H2H, rapidly fatal s Tx**	Bacteria in smear, gram stain	I- < 2500 worldwide foci; Africa esp DRC	Bubonic s Tx 50% pneumonic s Tx 100% streptomycin, gentamycin, doxycycline
Flies (gen F)						
Phlebotomus, et al (sandflies, F)	*Leishmania*	Cutaneous Leishmaniasis (CL) (Baghdad boil, Delhi boil, rose of Jericho)	Papule → nodule → <u>painless ulcer</u> occas c nodular lymphangitis, LN; CP of mucosal involvement (espundia) in New World disease	Amastigotes in stained slit skin smears; culture; Leishmanin test	I-1,000,000 worldwide foci; most in SA, Mediterranean, & ME-central Asia	Rare sodium stiboglu-conate (New World only)
Phlebotomus, et al (sandflies, F) [various mammals]	*Leishmania donovani et al* (Old World), *chagasi* (New World)	Visceral Leishmaniasis (VL) (kala-azar = black fever)	Most s Sx; F, LN, <u>massive HSM</u> → cirrhosis, pancyto-penia, dark skin at head & mouth (kala-azar); some c F, malaise, cough, D (// malaria); post-K-A dermal leish (PKDL) c diffuse papules & nodules at mouth, face, & trunk	Amastigotes in spleen > liver > BM > LN aspirate; serology	I-200 k-400 k worldwide foci; 90% in rural (sub)tropics of Brazil, Ethiopia, India, Somalia, S Sudan, Sudan	20–40,000 10% sodium stiboglu-conate

(continued)

Table 7.4.1b (continued)

Vectors [Reservoir]	Organism	Non-viral Diseases			Annual Incidence or Prevalence	Deaths/year or CFR Rx
		Name	Clinical	Lab Diagnosis		
Chrysops (deerflies, F)	*Loa loa*	Loiasis (Calabar swelling, African eyeworm)	Most s Sx; migratory Calabar swellings, pruritis, myalgia; CP of F, HA, meningism	Microfilariae in stained PS of noon spec	P-13,000,000 tropical SSA rainforest	0 DEC
Culicoides (biting midges, F)	*Mansonella*	Mansonelliasis	Most s Sx; transient itch, HA, arthralgia	Microfilariae in stained PS	SSA, LA	0 albendazole rarely needed
Simulium (blackflies, F)	*Onchocerca*	Onchocerciasis (river blindness)	Most s Sx; SC nodules, itch, rash (sowda, lizard skin, leopard skin), blindness	Microfilariae in skin Bx; if non-Dx, DEC challenge	P-18,000,000 300 k blind SSA >> LA riverine areas	0 ivermectin + albendazole
Glossina (tsetse flies, M & F) [humans—*Tbg*; cattle, game—*Tbr*]	*Trypanosoma brucei gambiense, rhodesiense*	African Trypanosomiasis (sleeping sickness)	Chancre (occas c hemor) → hemolymphatic stage—F, HA, local & occipital LN, SM → CNS stage—psyc Δs, sleep Δs, tremor, ataxia; *Tbr* > > *Tbg*	Tryps in stained PS, lymph, CSF; serology	I-500,000 W SSA *Tbg* E SSA *Tbr*	400,000 s Tx 100% s CNS suramin c CNS melarsoprol

Lice (M & F)						
Pediculus humanus (body, clothing lice) via feces, not directly via bite [humans] heavy clothing + poor sanitation = lice proliferation	*Bartonella quintana*	Trench Fever (Quintana fever)	F, malaise, HA, SM, shin pain, rash	BC; serology	Foci in Central Asia, LA, E & N Africa	0 doxycycline x 5 d; wash clothes at 50 °C or leave unworn x 1 wk
Pediculus humanus (body, clothing lice) via feces, not directly via bite [humans] heavy clothing + poor sanitation = lice proliferation	*Borrelia recurrentis*	Relapsing Fever (LBRF) (epidemic, louse-borne)	F 2–9 d alt s F 2–4 d c 1–3 relapses; assoc c HA, myalgia, NV, HSM, jaundice, petechial rash, Δ CNS; CP of nephritis, meningitis, myocarditis; **may be rapidly fatal s Tx**	Orgs in stained or darkfield PS	Foci in cold, rural, highland, temperate areas of Asia, E Africa, SA	s Tx 10% doxycycline x 5 d (JH in 90%); wash clothes at 50 °C or leave unworn × 1 wk

(continued)

Table 7.4.1b (continued)

Vectors [Reservoir]	Organism	Non-viral Diseases			Annual Incidence or Prevalence	Deaths/year or CFR Rx
		Name	Clinical	Lab Diagnosis		
Pediculus humanus corporis (body lice) via feces, not directly via bite [humans] heavy clothing + poor sanitation = lice proliferation	*Rickettsia prowazekii* **BW (B)**	Typhus Fever (LBTF) (epidemic, classic, jail fever, red louse disease) vector color indicative as bacteria multiply in gut & lyse epithelium → blood enters body cavity turning louse red; recrudescence years later = Brill-Zinsser disease	Malaise, myalgia 1–3 d → high F, C, HA, Δ CNS—delirium, stupor, coma, prostration, centrifugal rash d5 (central mac-pap → peripheral petechiae & purpura s face, palms, or soles), vasculitis c symmetric digital gangrene, strokes, shock, MODS; **rapidly fatal s Tx**; recrudescence gen short & mild	Serology—Weil-Felix reaction, IFA (gold standard)	Foci in cold, rural, highland, temperate areas of Asia (Russia), E Africa (Great Lakes, Ethiopia), SA (Peru); winter-spring; massive deaths in wars, famines, & migrations	s Tx 10–60% esp > 60 y/o c Tx < 5% doxycycline x 5 d (200 mg x1 dose in epidemics); wash clothes at 50 °C or leave unworn × 1 wk

Mites (M & F larvae)						
Leptotrombidium (trombiculid larval mites or chiggers) via saliva [rodents]	*Orientia* (prev *Rickettsia*) *tsutsugamushi*	Scrub Typhus (MBTF) (mite typhus, Tsutsugamushi fever)	Painless ulcer, eschar (distinguishes case from DDx of malaria, typhoid) → // LBTF + conjunctivitis, LN, HSM → vasculitis c DIC, ARF, MODS; **fatal s Tx** but lower mortality than LBTF	Serology—Weil-Felix reaction, IFA (gold standard)	Foci in scrub areas of S, SE Asia, Pacific islands; monsoon season	s Tx 1–30% gen < LBTF doxycycline
Liponyssoides	*Rickettsia*	Rickettsial Pox (vesicular rickettsiosis)	papule, LN; F, vesicular rash (s palms, soles)	Serology	E NA, Central Asia	Rare doxycycline
Mosquitoes (F)						
Anopheles	*Plasmodium falciparum, vivax, ovale, malariae*	Malaria (swamp fever)	*Pf* CP of cerebral malaria, ARDS, ARF (adults); **rapidly fatal s Tx**	Orgs in stained PS, RDT	I-200,000,000 #1 parasitic disease SSA, Asia, LA	438,000 90% in SSA nearly all U5 quinine, ACT
Culex, Anopheles, Aedes, et al	*Wuchereria bancrofti, Brugia malayi, timori*	Filariasis (lymphatic filariasis)	Most s Sx; *Wb* c recurrent F, LN, retrograde lymphangitis, lymphedema, TPE; CP of elephantiasis (limbs, breasts, genitals); *Bm, Bt // Wb* but F worse, CP only in distal exts	Microfilariae in stained PS of midnight spec, skin Bx; serology —Ag detection	P-110,000,000 S, SE Asia, SSA, LA P-13,000,000 S, SE Asia	0 albendazole + DEC or ivermectin (in oncho areas)

(continued)

Table 7.4.1b (continued)

Vectors [Reservoir]	Organism	Non-viral Diseases			Annual Incidence or Prevalence	Deaths/year or CFR Rx
		Name	**Clinical**	**Lab Diagnosis**		
Ticks (M & F)						
Ixodes (hard ticks in Ixodidae family eg deer ticks)	*Babesia*	Babesiosis	Most s Sx; F, C, malaise, myalgia, jaundice from HeAn, s rash	Orgs in stained PS	Worldwide foci	Clindamycin + quinine
Ixodes (hard ticks in Ixodidae family eg deer ticks)	*Borrelia burgdorferi*	Lyme Disease	Red papule → 1st stage (1–4 wks)—EM; 2nd stage (1–6 months)—F, HA, malaise, LN, EM (s palms & soles), neuro Sx (esp bilat Bell's), cardiac Sx (esp AVB), arthropathy (esp knees); 3rd stage (years)—episodic oligoarthritis, chronic myocarditis, polyneuropathy	Serology is inaccurate	NA, Eur, Asia; summer	Doxycycline
Ornithodoros (soft ticks in Argasidae family)	*Borrelia duttoni, et al*	Relapsing Fever (TBRF) (endemic, tick-borne)	// LBRF but milder (< HSM, jaundice, rash) c more relapses & longer course	Orgs in stained or darkfield PS	SSA (Somalia), ME, S Asia, NA, SA	s Tx < 2–10% doxycycline JH in 40%

Amblyomma, Ixodes (hard ticks in Ixodidae family)	*Ehrlichia*	Ehrlichiosis	F, C, HA, malaise, myalgia, sore throat s rash	Serology	USA, Japan not tropics	< 2% doxycycline
Dermacentor, et al (hard ticks in Ixodidae family eg wood ticks, dog ticks) via tick bite, aerosols from infected hosts, food contamination [rodents, lagomorphs]	*Francisella* **BW (A)**	Tularemia (rabbit fever)	Vector bite → local ulcer, regional LN; inhalation → F, C, HA, fatigue, pneumonia or sepsis; ingestion → pharyngitis, abd pain, DNV; **no H2H**	Serology at 2 wks		Rare s Tx 5–10% gentamycin
Amblyomma (hard ticks in Ixodidae family)	*Rickettsia africae*	African Tick Bite Fever	Multiple painless eschars, lymphangitis, LN, subtle rash // TBTF	Serology	SSA; people on safari	0 doxycycline

(continued)

Table 7.4.1b (continued)

Vectors [Reservoir]	Organism	Non-viral Diseases			Annual Incidence or Prevalence	Deaths/year or CFR Rx
		Name	Clinical	Lab Diagnosis		
Rhipicephalus sp. (hard ticks in Ixodidae family eg brown dog ticks)	*Rickettsia conorii* complex (multiple sero-types)	Tick-borne Typhus Fever (TBTF) (Mediterranean tick fever or spotted fever, boutonneuse fever, tick typhus of Kenya, Crimea, India, Israel)	Painless button eschar, LN, peripheral mac-pap rash d4 (palms, soles, & face)	Serology	Africa, India, Mediterranean	3–30% doxycycline
Dermacentor, et al (hard ticks in Ixodidae family eg dog ticks, wood ticks)	*Rickettsia rickettsii*	Rocky Mtn Spotted Fever (RMSF) (NA tick typhus, Sao Paolo fever, Tobia fever)	F, C, malaise, HA, myalgia, centripetal rash d5 (pink macules on palms, soles, & face → central petechiae)	Serology	E NA, LA; summer	s Tx 15–25% c Tx 3–5% doxycycline
> 40 tick species	None – neurotoxin	Tick Paralysis	Ascending, lower motor neuron paralysis c paresthesis → progressive c bulbar & resp paralysis	None – Dx is based on finding the tick; DDx Guillain-Barre	Worldwide foci; most in W NA, E Australia	Rare esp pedes <10 supportive Tx

Table 7.4.2
Tropical Infectious Diseases—Non-Vector-Borne

Hosts [Intermediate] Mechanism	Organism	Diseases			Annual Incidence or Prevalence*	Deaths/year or CFR Rx, Vaccine
		Group/name	**Clinical**	**Lab Diagnosis**		
		Bacteria				
	Actinomyces	Actinomycosis	Induration & draining sinuses in jaw, thorax (DDx fungi)	Orgs in gram stain	Worldwide sporadic	Ampicillin
Cats	*Bartonella henselae*	Cat-scratch Disease	Regional LN (10% suppurate); atypical presentations (5%) c lung or liver lesions, encephalitis, FUO	IFA; Bx	Worldwide	None azithromycin or none
Cattle, pigs, goats, sheep	*Brucella abortus, melitensis, suisi* **BW (B)**	Brucellosis (undulant fever, Malta fever)	Recurrent F, C, night sweats, lethargy, HA, arthralgia, visceral microabscesses, wt loss; CP of osteoarthritis, orchitis, endocarditis, meningitis	BC, BM culture; serology; PCR	Worldwide	s Tx 2% rifampicin + doxycycline

(continued)

Table 7.4.2 (continued)

Hosts [Intermediate] Mechanism	Organism	Diseases			Annual Incidence or Prevalence*	Deaths/year or CFR Rx, Vaccine
		Group/name	Clinical	Lab Diagnosis		
Environmental saprophyte [none—soil reservoir; animals may contract illness, but org is not zoonosis]	*Burkholderia pseudomallei* **BW (B)**	Melioidosis (Whitmore's disease, first described in Myanmar)	Most s Sx; bacteremia (60%) c sepsis, multiple abscesses, or typhoidal syndrome esp in ICPs or CIs; localized infection (40%) esp in lung (may look // TB), liver, spleen, skin → late reactivations	BC, UC, pus culture; serology	SE Asia, N Aus, SSA, LA; esp ICPs; rainy season	Ceftazidime; chloro + cotri + doxycycline
	Chlamydia	Trachoma	Conjunctival folliculitis → intense inflammation → scarring → trichiasis → corneal opacity → scarring → blindness	Orgs in epithelial cells of conj swab	P-150,000,000 2 m blind worldwide dry areas	SAFE c azithromycin, tetracycline ointment
	Clostridium	Tetanus	Onset 1 wk p injury; neonate—weakness, floppi-ness, irritability, inability to feed, spasms; adult—trismus, local & generalized spasms (4 prognostic classes)	None—Dx is clinical	I-1,000,000 pedes I-200,000	10–90% PCN + TIG

	Coryne-bacterium	Diphtheria	F, toxicity, tonsillopharyngitis c pseudomembrane & bleeding points, LN, neck edema; painful, cutaneous ulceration c palsy; CP of airway obstruction, myocarditis, HB			Non-cutaneous 5–10% procaine PCN + antitoxin
Sheep, cattle, goats, cats, dogs via airborne	*Coxiella burnetii* **BW (B)**	Q Fever (query fever)	Acute—F, C, malaise, HA, atypical pneumonia; chronic (< 1%)—FUO, granulomatous hepatitis c jaundice, endocarditis	Serology	Worldwide hot, dusty areas esp ranchers, livestock farmers	< 2% doxycycline, FQ
Cattle, other ruminants	*Escherichia coli* (6 pathotypes—ETEC, EHEC, EIEC, etc) **BW (B)**	Gastroenteritis (travelers diarrhea, shiga toxin-producing *E. coli*)	Acute DNV; dysentery if EHEC, EIEC; CP (5–10%) of HUS from EHEC O157:H7	SC	I-200,000,000 ETEC	380,000 ETEC mostlyU5 in DCs no vaccine

(continued)

Table 7.4.2 (continued)

Hosts [Intermediate] Mechanism	Organism	Diseases			Annual Incidence or Prevalence*	Deaths/year or CFR Rx, Vaccine
		Group/name	Clinical	Lab Diagnosis		
Rodents, pigs, cattle, dogs, raccoons via skin or MM	*Leptospira*	Leptospirosis (hemorrhagic jaundice, mud fever, rice field fever, canecutter's disease, swineherd disease, Weil's disease)	Anicteric syndrome (90%) (due to bacteremia)—F, C, HA, DNV, cough, conjuncti-vitis, rash, myalgia (lumbar & calf), malaise; myocardial, renal, liver disease (10%) → icteric syndrome (1%) (Weil's disease)—anicteric syndrome + HSM, deep jaundice, rash (orange skin), HeAn, purpura, GIB, HUS, ARF, AHF	Serology	Worldwide tropics c fresh water rivers, floods, or rainy season; esp farming, abattoir, sewer-age workers; riverine tourists	Weil's 10% doxycycline, PCN
	Neisseria meningitides (serogroups A, B, C W, Y)	Meningococcal Disease	Sepsis, meningitis, petechial rash; **rapidly fatal s Tx**	Orgs in CSF gram stain; BC, CSF culture	I-500,000 esp U5 worldwide; dry season epi-demics of group A in SSA	30–60,000 c Tx 10% ceftriaxone
	Salmonella enterica var Paratyphi (pathotypes A, B, C)	Paratyphoid Fever	// Typhoid F but milder—F, NVD (occas dysentery) c 10 d course; CP of bacteremia →bone, joints, GB, other organs (esp in SSD, HIV)	BC, SC	I- < < typhoid F	<< typhoid F FQ, ceftriaxone

	Salmonella enterica var Typhi **BW (B)**	Typhoid Fever (enteric fever, typhus abdominalis—confused c epidemic typhus thru 18th c)	Sustained or remittent F, C, malaise, fatigue, relative brady, HA, cough, myalgia, anorexia, N, abd pain, con-stipation, D, HSM, rose spots; CP of lower GIB (10%) & bowel perf (3%) from Peyer's patches, encephalopathy, meningitis, ARF, abscess	BC > SC wk 1 SC > BC wk 2+ UC, BM culture if above NG; Widal poor test but used in DCs	I-27,000,000 epidemic AR 6% P-2-5% infected chronically S Asia > > Africa	600,000 s Tx 10–20% c Tx < 1% highest CFR U5 FQ, ceftriaxone
	Shigella (4 species—*S. dysenteriae* type 1 (SD1) most severe, esp in emerg settings; *S. flexneri* most common in DCs; *S. sonnei* most common in ICs; *S. sonnei* & *S. boydii* c mild D) **BW (B)**	Shigellosis (bacillary dysentery)	F, NVD (initially watery, then small volume dysentery), anorexia, low abd pain, cramps, tenesmus, rectal prolapse (pedes); 25% will not have dysentery, but when present, it can last wks-months; CP (esp in SD1) of hypoglycemia, sepsis, encephalopathy, toxic megacolon, GI perf, HUS	SC, BC ID_{50} for SD1 = 10 SD1 (Shiga bacillus) produces Shiga toxin causing severest disease, longest duration of illness, higher ABX resistance, and highest CFR	I-175,000,000 esp U5, mal-nourished; endemic in Africa & Asia	1,000,000 mostly U5 s Tx 20% FQ

(continued)

Table 7.4.2 (continued)

Hosts [Intermediate] Mechanism	Organism	Diseases			Annual Incidence or Prevalence*	Deaths/year or CFR Rx, Vaccine
		Group/name	**Clinical**	**Lab Diagnosis**		
	Streptococcus	Rheumatic Fever	Major manifestations—carditis (mitral > aortic), polyarthritis (large joints), chorea, ery marginatum, or subcut nodules; minor manifestations—arthralgia, fever	Serology eg ASO titer. Dx is clinical (2 major or 1 major +2 minor) supported by Lx	I-300,000 P-15,000,000 developing countries; winter-spring esp adolescents	225,000 benzathine PCN
	Treponema pallidum pertenue	Yaws	3 phases—papilloma → frambesial lesions (wks-months); widespread esp palms & soles (months); destruction of skin & bone at exts (10% + of Pts) (5 years)		P-2500,000 tropics; esp pedes	Benzathine PCN, azithromycin

	Vibrio cholerae (O1 & O139 serogroups cause epidemics. O1 El Tor is cause of current (7th) pandemic. Other serogroups cause individual illness.) **BW (B)**	Cholera	Afebrile DNV c acute onset of <u>profuse</u>, <u>painless</u>, <u>rice-water stools</u>. No clinical differences between epidemic strains.	SC ID_{50} = 100,000+ 1st test is agglutination c O1 & O139 antisera. O1 serogroup divided into Inaba & Ogawa serotypes, plus classical & El Tor biotypes. All strains tested for CT—strains s CT do not cause epidemics.	I-2,800,000 worldwide; epidemic AR: 5% (refugees c malnut); 2% (rural under-served in non-endemic areas); 1% (WHO typical estimate of overall disease burden); 0.6% (endemic areas c poor sanitation)	100,000 s Tx 50% in severe disease c Tx < 1%

(continued)

Table 7.4.2 (continued)

Hosts [Intermediate] Mechanism	Organism	Diseases			Annual Incidence or Prevalence*	Deaths/year or CFR Rx, Vaccine
		Group/name	**Clinical**	**Lab Diagnosis**		
		Sexually Transmitted	**Bacteria and HSV**			
	Chlamydia trachomatis	Lymphogranuloma Venereum (LGV) (tropical bubo)	Single, small, painless, tran-sient genital ulcer → suppurative inguinal & pelvic LN (M c inguinal buboes, F c proctitis); CP of lymphedema, rectal stricture	IFA, PCR, culture of LN aspirate; serology	Worldwide esp tropics & subtropics	Rare doxycycline, erythromycin × 3 wks
	Haemophilus ducreyi	Chancroid (soft chancre)	Single or multiple deep, painful, necrotic, soft ulcers → painful, suppurative LN	Culture, IFA, PCR of exudate; serology	Worldwide esp inner city; M > F	0 ciprofloxacin x 3 d
	Herpes Simplex virus (HSV)	Herpes Simplex	Multiple painful vesiculo-pustular lesions → ulcers →systemic Sx c nonsuppurative inguinal LN → resolution	Dx gen clinical; Tzanck prep, viral culture of lesion	Worldwide	0 acyclovir
	Klebsiella (prev *Calymmato-bacterium*) *granulomatis*	Granuloma Inguinale (donovanosis)	Indurated papule → painless, beefy red ulcer c rolled edges → progressive ulceration & scarring c destruction of genitals → heme seeding to viscera & bone	Orgs in stained granulation tissue smear, Bx; PCR	Tropics & subtopics esp India, PNG, Caribbean	Rare doxycycline, erythromycin × 3 wks

	Treponema pallidum pallidum	Syphilis (lues)	1° – single, painless, firm chancre s LN (3 wks); 2° – mac-pap rash including palms & soles, generalized LN (6 wks); 3° – gummas (5 years), aortitis (10 years), meningitis (15 years). Pregnancy → still-birth (25%), neonatal death (15%), surviving syphilitic infant (40%)	Serology	12,000,000 worldwide	Benzathine PCN
	Treponema pallidum pallidum	Syphilis, congenital, early congenital	Congenital – LBW, feeding difficulty, bullous rash, jaundice, HSM; early congenital – NL at birth, but develops FTT, rash (3 months) // 2° syph c desquamation of palms & soles, saddle nose, nasal discharge, HSM	Serology	Developing countries	Benzathine PCN
			Mycobacteria			
	Mycobacterium leprae	Leprosy (Hansen's disease)	Hypopigmented/red skin patches c ↓/absent sensation (no itch or sweat) (≤ 5 patches = PB, > 5 patches = MB), peripheral nerve thickening; evolution of asymmetric tuberculoid disease → symmetric lepromatous disease; early CP of Type 1 reactions (skin and nerve inflammation), Type 2 reactions (ENL, F, malaise), silent NFI; late CP of iritis, osteitis, loss of digits	Orgs in AF stained slit skin smears ranging from PB to MB	P-650,000 S, SE Asia rural tropics	Rifampicin + dapsone + clofazimine + steroids (if CP)

(continued)

Table 7.4.2 (continued)

Hosts [Intermediate] Mechanism	Organism	Diseases			Annual Incidence or Prevalence*	Deaths/year or CFR Rx, Vaccine
		Group/name	**Clinical**	**Lab Diagnosis**		
	Mycobacterium tuberculosis	Tuberculosis (TB, consumption)	F, night sweats, wt loss, pulm Sx (85%), extrapulm Sx (15%)—LN (25%), pleurisy (25%), GU (15%), miliary (10%), bone (10%), CNS (5%), peritoneum (5%)	Orgs in AF stained sputum, body fluid, or tissue Bx; miliary orgs in liver Bx > transbronchial Bx > BM	I-10,000,000 MDR 500,000 P-17,000,000 infected 2 billion disease risk: s HIV 5–10% over lifetime; c HIV 10%/year	1,600,000 300,000 HIV+ 50% die/year RHZE if sensitive; refer if MDR
	Mycobacterium ulcerans	Buruli Ulcer	Painless, firm papule, nodule, or plaque (LE > UE) → ulcer c undermined edge → non-healing & extending	Orgs in AF stained smear	Worldwide tropics, SE Aus; esp pedes	Rifampicin + adjunct ABX; debridement or excision if wide ulcer
		Fungi				
		Subcutaneous				
	Madurella, Pseudallescheria, et al	Mycetoma (maduromycosis, Madura foot)	Painless, chronic subcut swelling, suppuration, & sinus tracts on extremities, esp foot; osteo	Org clusters (granules) in smear, histology	N Africa (Sudan), S Asia, CA; esp barefoot	Rare miconazole
	Phialophora, Fonsecaea, et al	Chromomycosis (chromoblastomycosis, dermatitis verrucosa)	Dark-pigmented, warty, ulcerated, & pruritic plaques on LE extending to con-tiguous tissues over years	Orgs in tissue Bx or scrapings; Bx culture	Tropical LA, SSA; agric workers esp barefoot	Rare itraconazole

	Sporothrix	Sporotrichosis	Nodules → painless ulcer (DDx CL, anthrax) → lymphocutaneous (70%) c nodular tracks on cordlike lymphatics	Culture of tissue Bx or pus; orgs rare on smear	Worldwide; esp farmers & gardeners	Rare itraconazole
		Systemic Fungi				
		Endemic Respiratory				
	Blastomyces	Blastomycosis (Gilchrist disease)	F, cough, pneumonia → chronic pulm disease → secondary spread c red papules, ulcers on face & distal exts	Orgs in unstained sputum smears	Worldwide; uncommon & sporadic	Itraconazole, amphotericin
	Coccidioides	Coccidioido-mycosis (San Joaquin fever, desert fever)	F, C, cough; rarely body abscesses in subcut tissues	Orgs in sputum smear, fluid, Bx	Arid USA, LA; uncommon	High in dis-seminated disease fluconazole, amphotericin
	Histoplasma capsulatum	Histoplasmosis	5 syndromes: no Sx; acute pulm; acute disseminated (F, LN, HSM, BM suppression); chronic disseminated; chronic pulmonary disease // TB c cavitation	Orgs in stained smears of body fluids	Worldwide foci in LA, USA, Africa, Asia, Aus	Itraconazole, amphotericin

(continued)

Table 7.4.2 (continued)

Hosts [Intermediate] Mechanism	Organism	Diseases			Annual Incidence or Prevalence*	Deaths/year or CFR Rx, Vaccine
		Group/name	Clinical	Lab Diagnosis		
	Histoplasma capsulatum var *duboisii*	Histoplasmosis Duboisii (African histoplasmosis)	Subacute, focal granuloma on skin, bone → secondary spread to skin, bone, LN, viscera	Orgs in stained smear of granuloma, tissue Bx	Africa	Itraconazole, amphotericin
	Paracoccid-ioides	Paracoccidioido-mycosis (S American blastomycosis)	Pneumonia c patchy infil-trates → mucosal ulcerations, LN; visceral involvement	Orgs in sputum smear, Bx; culture	Tropical LA; esp agric workers	Itraconazole, amphotericin
		Opportunistic Systemic				
	Aspergillus	Aspergillosis	Allergic bronchopulmonary aspergillosis; pulm asper-gilloma (fungus ball); cold skin abscesses; invasive end organ effects in brain, kidneys	Orgs in histology; culture	Worldwide; uncommon & sporadic ICPs	Itraconazole
	Candida	Candidiasis	F, end organ effects	Orgs in histology; culture	Worldwide; ICPs	Fluconazole amphotericin
	Cryptococcus	Cryptococcosis	Subacute-chronic meningitis esp in ICP; pneumonia	Orgs in stained CSF; serology	Worldwide; ICPs	Fluconazole amphotericin

	Pneumocystis jirovecii (prev *carinii*)	Pneumocystis Pneumonia (PCP) (plasma-cell pneumonia)	Pneumonia in ICP	Orgs in stained sputum, BAL, or lung Bx	Worldwide; ICPs	TMP/SMZ
	Rhizopus, et al (Mucoraceae)	Mucormycosis	Nasal or paranasal infection → craniofacial necrosis; blood vessel thrombosis c infarction of lung, gut	Orgs in tissue Bx; Bx culture	Worldwide; ICPs	Amphotericin
		Helminths				
		Nematodes				
		Intestinal Nematodes				
Humans via FO [none – geohelminth]	*Ascaris* (roundworm)	Ascariasis	Most s Sx; F, dry cough, wheeze (Loeffler's syn-drome); intestinal worms rarely noted; colicky abd pain, bowel obstruction, appendicitis, pancreatitis	Ova or worms in stool, sputum	P-1.5 billion tropics; esp pedes	Mebendazole, albendazole
Humans via FO [none]	*Enterobius* (threadworm, pinworm)	Enterobiasis	Most s Sx; perianal itch, anorexia, D	Ova on scotch tape swab (uncommon in stool)	P-350,000,000 esp pedes	Mebendazole, albendazole
Humans via skin of LE [none – geohelminth]	*Ancylostoma, Necator* (hookworm)	Ancylostomiasis, Necatoriasis	Most s Sx; ground itch, cutaneous larva migrans (esp c dog & cat hookworms), dry cough (// Loeffler's), abd pain, D, hypochromic anemia	Ova in stool (larvae in old specs)	P-900,000,000 women on agric plantation using nightsoil	50–60,000 mebendazole, albendazole

(continued)

Table 7.4.2 (continued)

Hosts [Intermediate] Mechanism	Organism	Diseases			Annual Incidence or Prevalence*	Deaths/year or CFR Rx, Vaccine
		Group/name	Clinical	Lab Diagnosis		
Humans via skin of LE [none—geohelminth]	*Strongyloides*	Strongyloidiasis	Triad of urticarial rash, abd pain (// PUD), D; also larva currens, dry cough (// Loef-fler's), dysentery; CP of hyperinfection syndrome c foul D, malabsorption, bowel perf, sepsis, encephalitis	Larvae in stool (ova uncommon unless D); duodenal aspirate; serology	P-60,000,000 co-existing c hookworm	Albendazole, ivermectin preferred
Humans via FO [none—geohelminth]	*Trichuris* (whipworm)	Trichuriasis	Most s Sx; abd pain, chronic dysentery, rectal bleeding & prolapse, anemia, malnutri-tion (trichuris dysentery syndrome)	Ova in stool; adult worm on sigmoidoscopy	P-500,000,000 tropics; esp pedes	Rare mebendazole, albendazole
		Filarial/Tissue Nematodes				
	Loa loa	See vector table—flies				
	Mansonella	See vector table—flies				
	Onchocerca	See vector table—flies				
	Wuchereria, Brugia	See vector table—mosquitoes				

		Zoonotic Nematodes				
Dogs, cats	*Ancylostoma* (dog, cat hookworm)	Cutaneous Larva Migrans (creeping eruption)	Reticulated subcutaneous track on foot or buttock	None		Albendazole, ivermectin
Rodents [snails]	*Angiostron-gylus*	Angiostrongyliasis (eosinophilic meningitis, visceral larva migrans)	Meningitis, eosinophilia	Often none; Hx of eating raw snails + meningitis + eos in PS, CSF; orgs in granuloma Bx	Asia-Pacific, LA tropics & subtropics	Mebendazole
[Marine fish]	*Anisakis*	Anisakiasis (visceral larva migrans)	Abd pain, NV, enteric abscesses, malaise	Orgs on endos-copy; tissue Bx; serology	Japan, Asia-Pacific, Scandinavia	Excision
Humans [none]	*Dracunculus* (Guinea worm)	Dracunculiasis	Blister on leg/foot, ulcer; emergence of worm	None	P-100,000 SSA c dry Climate	Extraction +/– ivermectin
Dogs, cats [freshwater fish]	*Gnathostoma*	Gnathostomiasis (visceral larva migrans)	Abd pain, NV, abd abscesses, malaise	Orgs in granuloma Bx; serology	SE Asia	Albendazole
[Freshwater fish]	*Onchocerca* (prev *Capillaria*)	Onchocerciasis (intestinal onchocerciasis)	Intermittent D, abd pain, malabsorption (protein losing), wt loss	Ova or larvae in stool	Philippines, Thailand	Rare but rapid metronidazole

(continued)

Table 7.4.2 (continued)

Hosts [Intermediate] Mechanism	Organism	Diseases			Annual Incidence or Prevalence*	Deaths/year or CFR Rx, Vaccine
		Group/name	**Clinical**	**Lab Diagnosis**		
Dogs, cats	*Toxocara canis, cati* (dog, cat roundworm)	Toxocariasis (visceral larva migrans)	Most mild & chronic; F, malaise, cough, broncho-spasm (// Loeffler's), HSM, LN, endophthalmitis	Orgs in granuloma Bx; serology	Worldwide; esp pedes	Albendazole
Pigs	*Trichinella*	Trichinellosis	F, myalgia, rash, periorb edema (// flu + facial edema); dry cough, myocarditis	Orgs in muscle Bx (classic spiral)	P-10,000,000	Albendazole
		Cestodes				
Humans, bears, foxes [cyclops → fish]:. foodborne	*Diphyllo-bothrium* (fish tapeworm)	Diphyllobothriasis	Most s Sx; D, megaloblastic anemia		P-10,000,000 Alaska, Canada	Praziquantel
Dogs [herbivores—sheep, cattle, pigs]	*Echinococcus granulosus* (dog tapeworm)	Echinococcosis (cystic or unilocular E, hydatid disease)	Most s Sx until enlarge; S/Sx referable to liver (70%), lung (20%), other organs (10%)	US, CT; serology	P-2,700,000 including *E. multilocularis* grazing countries where dogs eat viscera	2–5% albendazole + praziquantel excision p CT
Foxes, dogs, cats [rodents]	*Echinococcus multilocularis*	Echinococcosis (alveolar or multilocular E, hydatid disease)	Most s Sx until enlarge; S/Sx referable to liver, lung, brain; local invasion // tumor → death	US, CT; serology	P-as above N hemis—FSU, central Eur, N Japan, Alaska	s Tx 90% c Tx 20% surgery

Rodents [none]	*Hymenolepsis*	Hymenolepiasis (dwarf tapeworm)	Most s Sx; abd pain, D	Ova in stool	P-75,000,000 worldwide cities #1 human tapeworm in NA, LA	Praziquantel
[Cattle]	*Taenia saginata*	Taeniasis (beef tapeworm)	Most s Sx	Proglottid or ova in stool	P-77,000,000	Praziquantel
[Pigs]	*Taenia solium*	Taeniasis (pork tapeworm, cysticercosis)	Adult worm (from eating pig cysticerci)—anorexia, abd pain; larvae (from FO trans-mission of ova)—S/Sx referable to muscle, brain (epilepsy, HA, psyc), other organs	Proglottid or ova in stool; larvae in imaging & Bx; serology	P-10,000,000	Praziquantel
		Trematodes				
Fish [freshwater snails → fish]:. foodborne	*Clonorchis* or *Opisthorchis* (oriental liver fluke)	Clonorchiasis (Chinese liver fluke disease)	Anorexia, biliary colic, HM, cirrhosis, ascites, jaundice, cholangitis, CA	Ova in stool; serology	P-7,000,000 Asia	Praziquantel
Sheep, cattle [freshwater snails → plants] :. foodborne	*Fasciola hepatica* (liver fluke)	Fascioliasis	F, malaise, RUQ pain, biliary colic, HM, wt loss, jaundice, urticaria	Ova in stool; serology	P-2,000,000 worldwide	10,000 triclaben-dazole

(continued)

Table 7.4.2 (continued)

Hosts [Intermediate] Mechanism	Organism	Diseases			Annual Incidence or Prevalence*	Deaths/year or CFR Rx, Vaccine
		Group/name	**Clinical**	**Lab Diagnosis**		
Pigs [freshwater snails → plants] :. foodborne	*Fasciolopsis* (intestinal fluke)	Fasciolopsiasis	Anorexia, DNV	Ova in stool	P-15,000,000 SE Asia	Praziquantel
Dogs, cats, pigs [freshwater snails → crabs] :. foodborne	*Paragonimus* (lung fluke)	Paragonimiasis	Malaise, urticarial rash → chronic cough, hemoptysis, pleuritic chest pain	Ova in sputum or stool	P-20,000,000 worldwide foci China, Korea	Praziquantel
Humans (*Sm, Sh*); humans, dogs, cats, pigs, cattle, water buffalo, horses (*Sj*) [freshwater snails] :. percutaneous infection	*Schistosoma mansoni, hematobium, japonicum, et al* (blood fluke)	Schistosomiasis (bilharziasis, snail fever, Katayama fever)	F, urticaria, species specific Sx—terminal hematuria, obstructive uropathy (*Sh*); HSM, portal HTN, dysentery (*Sm*); Katayama F c urticaria, D, HSM, cough (4 wks p primary infection) (*Sj*)	Ova in stool (*Sm, Sj*), midday terminal urine (*Sh*); serology	P-200,000,000 Africa, SE Asia, SA 85% in SSA *Sh* > *Sm* > *Sj* > *Si* > *Smek*	200,000 praziquantel

		Invasive Ectoparasites				
Domestic, field hosts eg dogs, rats, humans (accidental) via direct contact with larva from eggs laid in soil or damp cloth	*Cordylobia* (tumbu fly, mango fly)	Myiasis	Boils	None	SSA	Topical petroleum jelly, forceps extraction
Via direct contact with fly eggs from vector or intermediate vector (eg housefly)	*Dermatobia* (bot fly)	Myiasis	Boils	None	LA	Excision
Via direct contact with adult mite	*Sarcoptes* (mite)	Scabies	Papules, burrows	Orgs on Px, micro	Worldwide	Permethrin
Domestic, field hosts via direct contact with adult flea	*Tunga* (jigger flea, sand flea)	Myiasis (tungiasis)	Pustules on toe webs	None	Worldwide tropics	Needle extraction

(continued)

Table 7.4.2 (continued)

Hosts [Intermediate] Mechanism	Organism	Diseases			Annual Incidence or Prevalence*	Deaths/year or CFR Rx, Vaccine
		Group/name	**Clinical**	**Lab Diagnosis**		
		Protozoa				
		Enteric				
	Balantidium	Balantidiasis	D (dysentery) NV, cramps, tenesmus	Trophs or cysts in wet or stained [stool]		Metroni-dazole + iodoquinol
	Cryptospo-ridium parvum **BW (B)**	Cryptosporidiosis	Chronic watery D esp in ICP	Oocysts in AF stained [stool]		50,000 none
	Cyclospora cayatanesis **BW (B)**	Cyclosporosis	Chronic watery D in ICP	Oocysts in AF stained [stool]		TMP/SMZ
	Entamoeba histolytica **BW (B)**	Amoebiasis	Most s Sx as ACPs; dysen-tery; liver abscess (gen s prior GI Sx, M > F)	Trophs or cysts in wet or stained [stool]; serology	I-50,000,000 P-500,000,000 tropics c poor sanitation	70,000 metronidazole + iodoquinol

	Giardia lamblia **BW (B)**	Giardiasis	Chronic watery D	Cysts or trophs in stained [stool]; string test	I-500,000,000	Metroni-dazole
	Isospora	Isosporosis	Chronic watery D in ICP	Cysts in AF stained [stool]		TMP/SMZ
		Non-Enteric				
Cats [sheep, goats, pigs, rodents, chickens]	*Toxoplasma gondii* **BW (B)**	Toxoplasmosis	Most s Sx; mono-like—F, LN; congenital triad of hydrocephalus, cerebral calcification, chorioretinitis; encephalitis & chorioretinitis in OD	Serology; PCR; orgs in tissue Bx	I-100,000,000 worldwide	300,000 pyrimeth-amine + sulfadiazine
	Trichomonas	Trichomoniasis	Mucosal discharge	Orgs in wet prep	I-175,000,000	0 metronidazole
		Viruses				
Via FO	Hepatitis A virus (HAV) **BW (B)**	Hepatitis A	F, malaise, anorexia, NV, RUQ pain, jaundice; no chronic infection	Serology	I-1,400,000	0.1–0.3% vaccine IG for PEP

(continued)

Table 7.4.2 (continued)

Hosts [Intermediate] Mechanism	Organism	Diseases			Annual Incidence or Prevalence*	Deaths/year or CFR Rx, Vaccine
		Group/name	Clinical	Lab Diagnosis		
Via sexual, perinatal, IDU, nosocomial	Hepatitis B virus (HBV)	Hepatitis B	F, malaise, anorexia, NV, RUQ pain, jaundice → acute fulminant (0.1–0.6%) c CFR 70%, chronic carriers (10%) → cirrhosis, HCC, hepatic failure	Serology	I-5,000,000 P-250,000,000 chronic carriers 2 billion infected worldwide 75% in Asia where P > 8%	< 1% 600,000 from Ca & cirrhosis vaccine HBIG for PEP
Via sexual, perinatal, IDU, nosocomial	Hepatitis C virus (HCV)	Hepatitis C	most s Sx → chronic carriers (80%) → cirrhosis, HCC, hepatic failure (// HBV)	Serology	P-200,000,000 80% chronic carriers most in Asia	50,000 no vaccine IG ineffective for PEP
Via sexual, perinatal, IDU, nosocomial	Hepatitis D virus (HDV)	Hepatitis D	F, malaise, anorexia, NV, RUQ pain, jaundice → chronic carriers → cirrhosis, HCC, hepatic failure	Serology	P-10,000,000	2–20% no vaccine IG, HBIG ineffective for PEP

Via FO esp water	Hepatitis E virus (HEV)	Hepatitis E	F, malaise, anorexia, NV, RUQ pain, jaundice; no chronic infections (// HAV)	Serology	I-20,000,000 3,000,000 acute cases epidemic AR 7%	57,000 < 1% unless pregnant, then 20% in 3rd tri no vaccine IG ineffective for PEP
Via sexual, perinatal, IDU, nosocomial	Human immuno-deficiency virus (HIV)	HIV/AIDS	Acute seroconversion over 1–2 wks c mac-pap rash (includes palms, soles), multiple Sx // mononucleosis; 4 stages—PGL → mild c mucocut Δs or HZ → intermediate c F, weight loss, chronic D → severe c AIDS, OIs	Serology	I-1,900,000 P-35,000,000 70% in SSA (5% of all adults in the region)	1,500,000 from TB, OD 70% in SSA ART trial vaccine
Via droplet nuclei	Influenza virus (types A, B, C; only A subtypes cause pandemic)	Influenza	F, HA, myalgia, malaise, nonproductive cough, sore throat, rhinitis	Virus isolation, IFA, RT-PCR, serology	I-5-10% non-pandemic	1,500,000 non-pandemic highest CFR U1 seasonal vaccine short-term antivirals

(continued)

Table 7.4.2 (continued)

Hosts [Intermediate] Mechanism	Organism	Diseases			Annual Incidence or Prevalence*	Deaths/year or CFR Rx, Vaccine
		Group/name	Clinical	Lab Diagnosis		
Via droplet nuclei	*Morbillivirus*	Measles	Cough, coryza, conjunctivitis, Koplik's spots, rash d3 x 4 d; CP of D, pneumonia, croup, deafness, brain damage	Serology	I-unknown SSA in cool, rainy season except Sahel where peaks in dry season	100,000 .1–5% in DCs; 10–30% in CEs c SAM vaccine
Via FO	Poliovirus (types 1, 2, 3; type 2 eliminated in wild in 1999)	Poliomyelitis (infantile paralysis)	Most s Sx (90–95%); F, HA, NV (4–8%); CP (< 1%) of myalgia, backache, asymmetric AFP LE > UE (0.1–0.5% c paralytic polio)	Virus isolation from stool; serology	I- < 100 endemic in Pakistan, Afghanistan, Nigeria	5–10% c paralytic polio polyvalent vaccine

* Disease incidence and prevalence estimates of chronic viruses and helminthes include subclinical infections for which asymptomatic carriers are common. For those infections, $P_{infection} > P_{disease}$

Reference

1. Yung A. Golden rules of infectious diseases. In: Yung A, McDonald M, Spelman D, et al. *Infectious diseases—a clinical approach*. 2nd ed. Hawthorne East, Victoria, Australia: IP Communications, 2005.

Document 7.5 EPIDEMIC PREPAREDNESS AND RESPONSE

I. EPIDEMIC PREPAREDNESS

A. Prior to Seasonal Epidemic

1. Establish a National Coordinating Committee (NCC).
2. Designate a lead agency and lead official in the NCC.
3. Establish a Local Coordinating Committee (LCC).
4. Designate a lead official in the LCC.
5. Anticipate roles for partner agencies (eg inter-agency and team coordination, disease surveillance, field epidemiological investigation, laboratory identification, case management guideline development, outbreak logistics, public information, and social mobilization).
6. Identify sources of funds.
7. Intensify disease surveillance.
8. Identify reference lab(s) for communicable diseases of epidemic potential.
9. Ensure mechanism for specimen transport.

II. OUTBREAK RESPONSE

A. Initial Response to Suspected Outbreak

1. Form an emergency team to investigate and manage the outbreak
   a. identify key roles on the outbreak investigation team(s)
      (1) epidemiology and surveillance
      (2) case management
      (3) water and sanitation
      (4) laboratory services
      (5) communication
   b. staff those roles
      (1) epidemiologist—to monitor proper data collection and surveillance procedures
      (2) physician—to confirm clinical S/Sx and train health workers in case management
      (3) water and sanitation expert—to develop a plan for reducing sources of contamination
      (4) microbiologist—to take environmental/biological samples for laboratory confirmation, train health workers in proper sampling techniques, and confirm use of appropriate methods in the diagnostic laboratory
      (5) behavior change communication (BCC) specialist—to assess the population's reaction to the outbreak, create, and disseminate appropriate health messages

B. Outbreak Investigation Protocol

1. Establish access, contacts, logistics.
2. Verify outbreak.
3. Confirm diagnosis.
4. Develop case definition.
   a. What are most patients complaining of?
   b. Describe a typical patient.
   c. Choose a case definition from the community descriptions confirmed by your own observations.
5. Count cases and determine demographic data.
   a. How many people live in the outbreak area?
   b. Who are the patients?
   c. What is their background—age, sex?
   d. Where are the patients coming from?
   e. When did the patients arrive?
   f. Why are the patients arriving?
   g. Count the number of patients fitting the case definition.
   h. Count the number of fresh graves or bodies at health facilities and inquire as to cause.
6. Orient the descriptive data—person, place, and time.
   a. Tabulate data on affected patients.
   b. Make a spot map.
      (1) When and where was/were the first reported case(s) seen indicating an outbreak?
   c. Plot an epidemic curve.
      (1) What is the present # of patients/day or week?
      (2) What is the usual # of patients/day or week?
      (3) Is this an increase?
      (4) What is the present # of deaths/week or month?
      (5) What is the usual # of deaths/week or month?
      (6) Is this an increase?
   d. Calculate attack rates and case fatality ratios for total patients, U5, O5, and gender.
7. Develop hypothesis.
   a. Postulate sources of disease and mechanism of spread.
   b. Estimate the population at risk of contracting disease and of dying from it.
      Consider especially:
      (1) poor
      (2) those with limited access to health services
      (3) minorities
      (4) malnourished
      (5) pregnant and lactating
      (6) infants not breast fed, children unvaccinated
      (7) elderly

8. Initiate control measures considering agent, host, and environment.
    a. What action has the community taken?
    b. Identify local response capacity.
        (1) What number and type of staff are locally available?
        (2) What drugs and supplies are locally available?
    c. Determine immediate unmet needs.
        (1) specimen collection and lab diagnosis
        (2) logistics
        (3) support for clinical care—staff, drugs, and supplies
        (4) support for environmental health
    d. Undertake further necessary actions.
        (1) case management with secondary prevention
        (2) patient isolation
        (3) health education
        (4) agent and reservoir identification
        (5) environmental decontamination
        (6) primary prevention
        (7) public information
9. Inform authorities with investigation report.
10. Initiate ongoing disease surveillance.

C. During Epidemic

1. NCC should meet at least weekly.
2. LCC should meet daily at first, then reduce meeting frequency as circumstances warrant.

D. Surveillance Systems Lessons Learned

1. Start small, keep it simple
    a. active surveillance at sentinel sites
    b. simple standard operating procedures
        (1) case investigation
        (2) specimen collection
2. Invest in local people and systems
3. Focus the system on performance-based indicators
    a. polio—non-polio acute flaccid paralysis detection rate of 1:100,000
    b. gastroenteritis—stool specimen collection rate of 80%
4. Link data to action
    a. case detection → local response
    b. case locations → need for (sub)national immunization days
    c. lab info → recognition of imported vs indigenous cases
    d. other process indicators → system improvement
5. Show success, then expand

Document 7.6
COMMUNICABLE DISEASE CONTROL

Glossary

ABX	antibiotics
AM	morning
AR	attack rate
ARI	acute respiratory infection
bd	twice daily
C&S	culture and antibiotic sensitivity
CFR	case fatality rate
CHW	community health worker
COTS	Cholera Outbreak Training and Shigellosis Program (training program developed at ICDDR)
CT	cholera toxin
d	day(s)
D	diarrhea
DF	dengue fever
DOC	drug of choice
Dx	diagnosis
EHEC	enterohemorrhagic *E. coli*
EPI	Expanded Programme on Immunization
ETEC	enterotoxigenic *E. coli*
F	fever
h	hour(s)
HPI	history of present illness
HUS	hemolytic-uremic syndrome
ICDDR	International Centre for Diarrhoeal Disease Research, Bangladesh
ID_{50}	median infective dose
IPD	inpatient department
IPT	intermittent preventive treatment
IRS	indoor residual spraying
ITN	insecticide treated net
IV	intravenous
IVF	intravenous fluids
L	liter
LCC	Local Coordinating Committee
MOH	Ministry of Health
N	nausea
N/A	not available
NCC	National Coordinating Committee
NGT	nasogastric tube
O5	over 5 year-old
OCV	oral cholera vaccine

OPD	outpatient department
ORS	oral rehydration salts/solution
p	person
PO	by mouth
PPE	personal protective equipment
PRN	as needed
Pt(s)	patient(s)
P_T	population total
q	every
qd	daily
rBS	recombinant beta subunit (of cholera toxin)
RDT	rapid diagnostic test
SD1	*S. dysenteriae* type 1
SMC	seasonal malaria chemoprophylaxis
SSU	short stay unit
S/Sx	signs and symptoms
STEC	Shiga toxin producing *E.coli*
Sx	symptoms
T	temperature
U2	under 2 year-old
U5	under 5 year-old
V	vomiting
WHO	World Health Organization
YF	yellow fever
yr	year(s)
Zn	zinc

Contents

This Annex profiles selected communicable diseases of epidemic potential whose incidence, management complexity, or mortality obliges particular attention.

- Diarrhea
- Influenza
- Malaria
- Measles
- Meningitis
- Viral Hemorrhagic Fever

The profiles are structured to quickly orient field staff to key issues in:

- Pathogens
- Epidemiology
- Preventive Medicine
- Epidemiological Surveillance
- Clinical Medicine
- Epidemic management

DIARRHEA

Pathogens

Cholera

V. cholerae has >200 serogroups. Serogroups are classified by biotype, and for serogroup O1, by serotype and biotype. Humans are the only known vertebrate host for cholera, and only serogroups O1 and O139 cause epidemic disease. There is no clinical difference between them. Other serogroups may cause disease in individuals, but not epidemics. When a suspected cholera serotype (strain) is isolated in the lab, one of the first tests performed is bacterial agglutination with O1 and O139 antisera. Strains are thereby identified as *V. cholerae* O1, O139, or non-O1/non-O139.

- If (+) agglutination to O1 antisera, then the strain is further tested for agglutination to antiserum of Ogawa and Inaba serotypes.
- If (+) agglutination to O139 antisera, then the strain is not further subdivided (except as producer or non-producer of CT as noted below).
- If (−) agglutination to O1 and O139 antisera, then the strain is known as non-O1, non-O139 *V. cholerae*.

A strain is further identified as a producer or non-producer of cholera toxin (CT). CT production is a major determinant of disease development. Strains lacking CT do not produce epidemics even if from the O1 or O139 serogroup.

- Serogroup O1 exists as 2 main biotypes—classical and El Tor—though hybrids also exist. Each biotype occurs as two serotypes—Ogawa and Inaba. Classic biotype caused the 5th and 6th pandemics but little epidemic disease since the 1970s though it still causes cases in India. **El Tor biotype** caused the 7th (current) pandemic and almost all recent outbreaks. El Tor was first isolated in 1905 in El Tor, Egypt after importation by Indonesian pilgrims travelling to Mecca. It survives longer in the environment and produces CT similar to the classical biotype. Presumably because of CT pathogenicity, the % of cholera patients with severe disease has doubled over the past 10 yrs. These patients tend to require IV fluid therapy.
- Serogroup O139 may have evolved from strains of O1 El Tor as they share many properties though not agglutination. In spring of 2002 in Dhaka, O139 cases exceeded O1 El Tor cases for the first time, and it was postulated that O139 may become the cause of an 8th pandemic. However, since then, O1 has again become dominant.

Infective dose depends on individual susceptibility. Relevant host factors include immunity produced by prior infection with serogroup O1 as well as stomach acidity. ID_{50} may be 100,000 orgs, so personal hygiene plays a lesser role than in shigellosis where the ID_{50} is much lower.

Shigella

Shigella has 4 species.

- *S. dysenteriae* type 1 (SD1 or Shiga bacillus) causes the severest disease of all *Shigella* sp because of its neurotoxin (Shiga toxin), longer duration of illness, higher ABX resistance, higher CFR thru invasive complications, and great epidemic potential.
- *S. flexneri* is the most common, and is generally endemic, in developing countries
- *S. sonnei* is the most common in industrial countries
- *S. boydii* and *S. sonnei* give mild disease.

Table 7.6.1
Shigella Species

Species	Serogroup	Serotypes	Notes
S. dysenteriae	A	1–15	SD1 gives most severe disease with complications of HUS
S. flexneri	B	1–6 (15 subtypes)	Greatest burden of disease and main cause of endemic shigellosis
S. boydii	C	1–18	Mild disease
S. sonnei	D	1	Mild disease

ID_{50} may be 10 orgs, so personal hygiene plays a greater role than in cholera.

E coli

Some kinds of *E. coli* produce a Shiga toxin. Shiga toxin genes reside in a bacteriophage genome integrated into the bacterial chromosome. Some ABX, eg fluoroquinolones, induce expression of phage genes. The bacteria that make these toxins are variously called "Shiga toxin-producing *E. coli*" (STEC), "enterohemorrhagic *E. coli*" (EHEC), or "verocytotoxic *E. coli*" (VTEC). All terms refer to the same group of bacteria.

- *E. coli* O157:H7 (often called "*E. coli* O157" or "O157") is the most commonly identified STEC in North America, and it causes most *E. coli* outbreaks. Approximately 5–10% of EHEC infections result in HUS.
- Non-O157 STEC serogroups also cause disease. In the USA, serogroups O26, O111, and O103 are the most commonly identified *E. coli* pathogens overall.

Epidemiology

Diarrhea epidemiology is seasonally dependent. Environmental temperature directly influences biologic activity—Δ5 °C is proportional to 3× risk of disease

- temperate climates: bacterial diarrhea in warmer, humid season; rotavirus diarrhea in cooler, dry season
- tropical climates: bacterial diarrhea in rainy season; rotavirus diarrhea year round with increased incidence in cooler season
- most common pathogens for watery diarrhea—rotavirus, ETEC, *V. cholerae*; most important pathogen for epidemic watery diarrhea—*V. cholerae*
- most common pathogens for dysentery—shigella species, salmonella species, *Campylobacter jejuni*, *Clostridium difficuile*, EIEC, EHEC, *E. coli* O157:H7, *Entamoeba histolytica*, *Yersinia enterocolitica*; most important pathogens for epidemic dysentery—*S. dysenteriae* serotype 1 (developing countries), *E. coli* O157:H7 (developed countries)

Bangladesh has 2 seasonal cholera peaks: pre-monsoon with hot, humid weather (esp weeks 15–20 in Apr-May) creating increased biological activity; post-monsoon (esp weeks 30–40 in Aug-Sep) with contamination of water sources. Pre-monsoon epidemics are generally worse than post-monsoon ones. Dysentery has low level year-round incidence, but epidemics occur roughly each decade. Epidemic strains display new, additive antibiotic resistance which probably triggers the epidemic. Once resistant strains have become endemic, antibiotic susceptibility rarely reappears. SD1 acquires resistance quickly. *Sf* acquires it more slowly, and that resistance may wane with decreasing ABX pressure.

At ICDDR, annual proportional incidence approximates the following:

Table 7.6.2
Proportionial Incidence of Diarrheal Pathogens in Bangladesh

Total		Pedes	
Rotavirus	30%	Rotavirus	45%
Cholera (O1 > > O139)	20%	*E. coli*	45%
ETEC	15%	Camplyobacter	10%
Shigella (flexneri > > boydii, sonnei, SD1)	5%		
Other	30%		

- *E. coli* overall = 35% of cases, but ETEC = 15%.
- *E. coli* tends to dominate before monsoon season and flooding
- Cholera tends to dominate after monsoon season and flooding
- Overall, 60–70% of diarrhea cases may be vaccine-preventable.
- 30% of Pts have no pathogen identified.

Preventive Medicine

Clean water and waste management especially for cholera.

Personal hygiene (hand washing with soap and clean towels) especially for shigella.

Water safe drinking water (boiled, chlorinated)

NB Sphere standards are not enough—you need increased quantities of chlorinated water at household level.

San clean latrines for safe disposal of excreta

hand washing with soap

Food safe food (cooked, stored)

breast feeding

Fomites safe disposal of dead bodies with disinfection of clothing

NB After outbreak of a fecal-oral pathogen, food hygiene and funereal practices may influence human-to-human transmission more than water quality.

Health education to affected population

Wash hands with soap:

after using toilets/latrines.

after disposing of children's feces.

before preparing food.

before eating.

before feeding children.

Boil or disinfect water with chlorine solution. (Bottle it, boil it, ferment it, or forget it.)

Eat only freshly cooked food. (Peel it, cook it, or leave it.)

Do not defecate near water sources.

Use latrines and keep them clean.

Consider vaccination for areas and populations most at risk. Pre-emptive vaccination for new arrivals (esp nutritionally impaired IDPs) moving into an endemic area is increasingly accepted. Reactive vaccination where cholera has broken out is more controversial—particularly if vaccine stocks are not locally available and remain limited worldwide. There are 2 types of oral cholera vaccines licensed internationally: one with dead *V. cholerae*, and one with live *V. cholerae*. (Parenteral cholera vaccine is not recommended because of low protective efficacy and frequent severe adverse reactions.)

killed whole cell *V. cholerae* O1 vaccine

- Dukoral—mixture of the classical biotype (both Inaba and Ogawa serotypes) and the El Tor biotype (only Inaba serotype) + purified recombinant B-subunit of CT (rBS)

  Dose: 3 cc vaccine given in 150 cc of buffer solution; 2 doses, 1–6 wks apart; cold chain required. The regime is identical for all patients, and thus can't be given to pedes <2 yr because of volume loading.

Dukoral has been the main vaccine considered for use in high-risk populations.

- mORC-VAX and Shanchol—similar to Dukoral except they do not contain the rBS, hence do not require a buffer, and are 1/3 the cost to produce. mORC-VAX, produced in Vietnam, is derived from a vaccine administered to millions of people since 1997, but is not WHO pre-qualified, and is not expected to have international distribution.
- Shanchol, produced in India, has international distribution (eg used in the Haiti cholera vaccination campaign of 2012), and is now the agent of choice for WHO. It confers immunity 10d p 2nd dose, effectiveness > 85% at 6 mo, and protection >50% at 5 yr. Also confers short-term protection vs ETEC.

  Dose: 1.5 cc vaccine followed by water ingestion but no fasting needed; 2 doses, 2 wks apart; cold chain required except for day of use.

live-attenuated genetically modified *V. cholerae* O1 vaccine

- Orochol—bivalent formulation as in Dukoral without rBS of CT.

  Dose: single dose. No longer manufactured.

WHO recommendations: "Vaccination should not disrupt the provision of other high-priority health interventions to control or prevent cholera outbreaks. Vaccines provide a short-term effect that can be implemented to bring about an immediate response while the longer term interventions of improving water and sanitation, which involve large investments, are put into place." [1]

ICDDR recommendations: "Because of limitations in terms of transport, formulation, and cost of the current Dukoral vaccine, the COTS program does NOT require the utilization of the vaccine during an outbreak; it is NOT necessary to vaccinate to overcome an outbreak. However, if Dukoral is readily available and staff are properly trained in its use according to the guidelines that come with the vaccine, the COTS program PERMITS Dukoral's use (ideally before an outbreak) in the following high-risk populations: refugee populations in which cholera is present, health care workers managing cholera cases, and communities in which the incidence rate is greater than 1 in 1000 annually." [2]

Epidemiological Surveillance (specific to cholera)

Cholera

Epidemiological assumptions (WHO, COTS):

Estimated attack rates:	10–20% extremely vulnerable hosts and poor environmental health (WHO)
	5% (refugee camps with malnutrition) (COTS)
	2% (rural communities of <5000 p) (COTS)

	1% (severe epidemic—good estimate of ultimate disease burden) (WHO)
	0.6% (endemic areas with bad sanitation) (COTS)
	0.2% (endemic areas in open settings—suitable for initial calculations of early resource requirements)
	NB Overall, 90% of cases are mild and difficult to distinguish from other types of D.
	NB Asymptomatic carriers are very common (10x # of cases).
Referral rates for IVs	20% of cases (much higher—70% at ICDDR as it shortens recovery time)
Case fatality ratios	1% (with good care)

The following catchment populations will yield 100 acute Pts of whom 20 will be severely dehydrated:

refugee camp of 2000 people (AR of 5% = 100 Pts)
open settings in endemic area with 50,000 people (AR 0.2% = 100 Pts)

A population of 100,000 infected individuals in an epidemic area will yield the following (WHO):

Population infected	100,000
Clinical cases	1,000 (1% of infected population)
Cases needing early resources	200 (20% of cases)
Cases needing IV therapy	200 (20% of cases)
Anticipated deaths	10 (1% CFR)

NB In non-endemic areas, AR adults > AR pedes because adults have higher exposure risks.
In endemic areas, AR pedes > AR adults because adults have been exposed since childhood

Clinical Medicine

Delivery of Health Services

Active case finding through CHWs
Treatment facilities—2 types

outpatient ORS center

1. ORS packets, Zn
2. clean water
3. ABX (in the case of a shigellosis outbreak)
4. recording form for demographic information
5. trained staff (nurse, health aides)
6. soap to give to families (especially in the case of a shigellosis outbreak)

7. communication (radio, telephone) with the treatment facility for patients who need transfer, and means of transport (ambulance, horse, rickshaw, etc.)

inpatient treatment facility (section of existing hospital/health center or makeshift facility)

1. one way traffic flow—from triage to OPD/home and IPD
2. running water or close proximity to water source
3. large quantities of safe water (40–60 L/p/d)
4. adequate waste disposal system
5. shelter from weather
6. recording form for patient demographic information and clinical status
7. IVs, suspension lines, ORS, meds, and other essential supplies in treatment areas
8. trained staff including physicians, nurses, health aides, and cleaners with supervision of Pts 24/7
9. fee waiver policy for emergencies
10. 1 family carer or visitor/Pt

Standardized Case Management

Suspected cholera outbreak definition

Pt > 5 yr develops acute watery diarrhea with severe dehydration or death

any sudden increase in the daily # of patients with acute watery diarrhea especially if they pass typical rice-water stools

Case definitions

cholera

where the disease is not known to be present:

Pt > 5 yr with acute watery diarrhea plus severe dehydration or death

where the disease is confirmed present:

Pt > 2 yr with acute watery diarrhea

bacillary dysentery

Pt with acute diarrhea plus visible blood in the stool

Treatment protocols

Overview

assess for dehydration

rehydrate the Pt

maintain hydration by replacing ongoing fluid losses until diarrhea stops

give an oral antibiotic to the Pt with severe dehydration

feed the Pt

Triage by dehydration status

1/3 Pts without dehydration → OPD for ORS

2/3 Pts with dehydration → SSU for IVF, ORS

→ IPD for adults with D > 14d, typhoid fever, meningitis; pedes with malnutrition + infectious complications

HPI & stool appearance help make presumptive Dx

Shigella HPI: 3 d of Sx with F + abdominal pain/cramps + bloody D (not voluminous) + tenesmus (from colonic mucosal inflammation and erosions), anorexia ± dehydration.

Stools: chunky style with visible coagulated blood (related to coagulation necrosis in bowel). However, watery diarrhea may appear early in the illness.

Cholera HPI: 6 h of Sx onset in early morning with V, profuse watery D without pain or cramps, marked dehydration.

Stools: homogeneous rice water, occasionally turbid with fine particulate, occasionally yellowish when mixed with urine.

Vibrio parahemolyticus

Stools: "meat-washed stool" treated similar to cholera

Rotavirus

HPI: V without F

Stools: look like mashed pulses

Amoeba Stools: appears dark brown because the parasite oxidizes heme.

IVF ASAP (< 1 minute) if severely dehydrated. 75 + % of Pts with dehydration at ICDDR get IVs because they feel better more quickly. Otherwise PO sufficient. NGT ok if IV and PO are unsuccessful (very rare).

NB: acetate in cholera saline may cause hypocalcemia and tetany.

ORS for rehydration

Pt < 6 months, glucose ORS

Pt > 6 months, rice-based ORS

Zn Pt < 6 months, 10 mg PO qd × 10–14 d

Pt > 6 months to 5 yr, 20 mg PO qd × 10–14 d

ABX always given under physician supervision

avoid prophylactic use

Cholera

In epidemic season, use ABX x 1 dose with all dehydrated patients with suspected cholera.

In non-epidemic season, use clinical judgment on watery diarrhea.

If organism is sensitive, doxycycline is generally DOC. ICDDR has used azithro as DOC in all ages.

Dysentery

Use ABX for dysentery year round (if resources limited, prioritize high risk groups—U5, malnourished, toxic, post-measles, pregnant, old, etc). If organism is sensitive, cipro is generally DOC. ICDDR has used cipro in adults and pivmecillinam in pedes. Ceftriaxone is 2nd choice for both age groups.

Rotavirus

No ABX unless Pt is very ill and clinical picture suggests combined disease.

ETEC

Usually, no ABX, unless Pt develops severe dehydration.

Misc Sx Vomiting: no antiemetics, but use NGT or IVF if Pt ultimately can't take PO

Fever: ± antipyretics depending upon resources available

Physician rounds q 2 h on severely ill Pts; 4x/d on Pts with some dehydration (SSU); 2x/d on Pts without dehydration (OPD).

Disposition

Cholera improves quickly—young Pts get off IVF by 24 h, old Pts by 48 h.

ETEC lasts for 3–5 d.

Shigella dysentery lasts for 3–5 d if uncomplicated.

Rotavirus lasts for 5 d until kids can feed again (strips off brush border). Maternal motivation is important during this time.

Overall, rice-based ORS ends up adequately treating 85% of diarrheas.

Discharge

no dehydration, < purging, able to take ORS adequately

5–7% return visits are expected; > 10% return visits mean discharge policy is too aggressive

<u>Essential drugs & supplies</u>

- cholera kits
- drug choices driven by culture data (10–20 specs)

<u>Referral guidelines</u>

- refer all Pts refractory to rehydration and standard ABX to hospital for definitive care

<u>Secondary prevention for the patient</u>

- ORS liberally distributed with instructions for use—2 ORS sachets to all discharged Pts (home based salt solution is dangerous)
- soap distribution to accompanying persons

<u>Secondary prevention at the site</u>

- isolate the affected Pt/ward/camp/defecation area.
- impose hand washing upon entry/exit to affected hut/clinic/camp/defecation area, etc (0.05% Cl).

in-service staff—HCWs should not handle food or water (ORS); kitchen staff should not handle hospital waste.

- recruit cleaners, establish cleaning routine (0.5% Cl).
  - wash spills ASAP
  - wash floor q 4 h
  - collect stool collection buckets bd or PRN (wash them with 2.0% Cl)
  - change and wash cot covers qd
  - wash cots after each Pt
  - spray the affected area qd (water storage containers, water distribution points, latrines, door handles, etc in clinic, camp, and defecation area)
- identify body fluid disposal site (2.0% Cl).
  - hold Cl treated fluids 2 h before dumping
- establish hygienic funereal practices (2.0% Cl)

Epidemic Management

<u>Outbreak investigation protocol in place</u>

- rapid response teams to investigate case reports
- epidemic investigation kits to mobilize
- specimens to collect
- labs to confirm Dx of *V. cholerae*, *S. dysenteriae*, other shigella, and *E. coli* O157:H7
  - dipstick identification on representative sample of specs is useful for cholera, but C&S is essential because dipsticks are not available for shigella, ETEC. Vibrio are hardy if kept moist and cool. They can survive a week in Cary Blair media. Shigella are fragile and difficult to recover if transport time > 1 d.
  - 5–10 isolates initially to confirm outbreak
  - 30–50 isolates initially to create ABX use policy (bacterial resistance renders cotrimoxazole, amp/amox, nalidixic acid, and tetracycline unusable)
  - 20–30 isolates monthly from IPD and OPD before ABX therapy to assess evolving ABX resistance
  - 10–20 isolates periodically to reference laboratory to confirm ABX resistance patterns and undertake molecular studies
  - 20 isolates at end of the outbreak to confirm that new diarrheas are not epidemic pathogens

NB Systematic sampling is most representative—eg every 10th Pt or all Pts q 2 weeks adjusted as needed to collect the necessary specs.

Sensitivity > > important than specificity in RDT screening during an epidemic.

Pts from one geographic area are more likely to constitute a cluster involving a new pathogen.

An area may be considered cholera-free after 2 incubation periods (total of 10 d) have passed without cholera disease. However, hospital monitoring should continue for a year due to tendency of enteric pathogens to re-emerge long after they are declared gone.

Cholera may be viable but nonculturable from the environment; environmental monitoring has many false negatives.

consider improvements to existing diagnostic labs

- hotline set up for reporting of rumor

Health reference and educational materials in place

- case definitions
- case management and referral guidelines for communicable diseases with epidemic potential
- Pt, provider, and community educational materials
- specimen handling protocols

Epidemic command & control center established

- principles and practices of incident mgmt
- unified command of multi-disciplinary specialists
- information channel to government and stakeholders
- support by government for technical actions

Coordination with technical sectors—particularly WASH (CFR is a function of case mgmt, but AR overall is a function of WASH)

- water supply, purification, and distribution systems
  - bucket chlorination is low tech but reasonable way to reach individual HH or small communities
  - water treatment units need Ca hypochlorite, chlorimetric, and colimetric monitoring devices
  - chlorinators worth considering at water sources of high public demand and epidemic activity
- hygiene promoters with environmental health assessors to address hand and food hygiene in communities around the outbreak area (think ring vaccination with knowledge)safe disposal of medical waste and infectious sludge from treatment facilities

Medical logistics—resource prepositioning and stockpiles

- cots (take one and have carpenter make copies)
- plastic sheets with defecation hole or sleeve
- buckets (white color for stool—enables recognition of diarrhea color; different color for emesis; different color for domestic waste)
- IVF, IV sets, IV poles or suspension cords (cholera kits)
- ORS powder and ORS vats (> 50 L)
- cups, spoons
- NGTs, syringes
- soap, cleaning supplies
- bleaching powder (eg Ca hypochlorite)—chlorinate water sources where feasible, otherwise bucket chlorinate at untreated sources
- equipment (eg chlorimetric and colimetric monitors)

Information management

- update local authorities
- intensify disease surveillance (health authorities, WHO)
- issue health advisories (health & political authorities)
- reinforce training of public health cadres on diarrhea prevention and control
- reinforce education of clinicians on diarrhea case management and secondary prevention
- initiate public awareness and health education campaign
  - health messages content (WHO Cholera manual or COTS card for Health Promotion Worker)
  - health messages dissemination—printed, loudspeaker, broadcast, community groups
  - health messages uptake—community understands hand washing, ORS use, and 2 prevention measures

OCV

- Cholera epidemic brings huge political pressures to DO something. This often translates into a hastily conceived vaccination campaign that distracts from core principles of cholera management. For every symptomatic Pt, there may be 90 asymptomatic carriers. In an established epidemic, the affected community is already extensively infected. Cholera vaccination, under these circumstances, has little public health benefit for the resource investment. If undertaken, the following will apply:
- Vaccination campaign requires numerous staff. Community mobilizers are key. Clinical staff should not be poached from their clinical duties. Supervisors must be free to move at will.
- Logistics is key—if the 1st day goes badly, the campaign goes badly.
- Mark the domiciles which are done.
- Hold after-action meetings each day.
- Last day, use mobilizers with mobile broadcasting to attract those who missed out.
- Second phase vaccination should include CHWs with multi-purpose messages on water and sanitation.

Key lessons in epidemic

Avoid: press exaggeration
ABX prophylaxis
reliance on IVF and insufficient ORS
lab investigation of cases once epidemic etiology is ascertained
prolonged hospitalization
hospital discharge criteria requiring multiple negative stool cultures
enthusiasm for OCV during epidemic
exaggerated water purification objectives
concentration of technical competencies in MOH at expense of districts
failure to share information with stakeholders

References

1. World Health Organization. Cholera vaccines: WHO position paper. *Weekly Epidemiological Record* 26 March 2010; 85(13):117–28.
2. International Centre for Diarrhoeal Disease Research, Bangladesh, and Swiss Tropical Institute (eds). Cholera outbreak training and shigellosis (COTS) program [CD-ROM version 1.0, undated]. Available from: International Centre for Diarrhoeal Disease Research, Bangladesh, and http://www.cotsprogram.com.

INFLUENZA

Pathogens

Influenza viruses comprise 3 genera—influenza types A, B, and C—each with 1 species.

- Influenza type A is divided into subtypes based upon serological response to hemagglutinin (HA) and neuraminidase (NA) glycoproteins. There are 16 different HA subtypes and 9 different NA subtypes. H1N1, H2N2, and H3N2 are responsible for the major human pandemics in the last century. H2N2 virus circulated between 1957 and 1968 but currently does not. Only influenza A subtypes infect birds, and all subtypes can do so. Bird flu viruses do not usually infect humans. But, in 1997, an outbreak of H5N1 avian influenza in poultry in Hong Kong marked the first known direct human transmission of avian influenza virus from birds to humans. Since then, H5, H7, and H9 avian influenza subtypes have been shown to infect humans.
- Influenza type B is morphologically similar to A and also creates seasonal and epidemic disease.
- Influenza type C is rare but can cause local epidemics.

Seasonal human influenza vaccine currently has 3 strains—H1N1/H3N2/B.

Influenza disease in humans has a short incubation period (1–3 d). Early symptoms are non-specific. It is highly infectious, especially early in the course of the disease, with a large # of asymptomatic carriers. Transmission potential (R_0) is a function of infectivity, period of contagiousness, daily contact rate, and host immunity. In general, the faster the transmission, the less feasible is interrupting transmission thru usual disease control tools of case finding, isolation, contact tracing, and ring vaccination.

Table 7.6.3
R_0 of Different Diseases (adapted from CDC [1])

Disease	R_0
Influenza pandemic	2–3 (1918)
Influenza seasonal	1.5–3
Measles	12–18
Polio	5–7
Rubella	6–7
Diphtheria	6–7
Smallpox	5–7
Mumps	4–7
SARS	3 (excluding superspreaders)

Table 7.6.4
Disease Comparison (adapted from US DHHS [2])

Attribute	Disease		
	Influenza	**Smallpox**	**SARS**
Transmissibility	High	Medium	Low
R_0	> 2 (estimated 1.8 for 1918 pandemic)	5–7	3 (excluding superspreaders)
Geography	Widespread, multi-focal epidemics		Focal epidemics
Transmission location	Community		Within families and health care settings
Incubation period	1–3 days	10–12 days (CDC)	7–10 days
Attack rate	10–35%	58% (CDC)	low
CFR	1% (seasonal) 50% (highly pathogenic avian influenza)	50% (unvaccinated) 30% (vaccinated post exposure) 11% (> 20 y before exposure) 1.4% (0–10 y before exposure)	5–10%
Epidemic investigation	Unlikely to track spread based upon movement of infected persons or contacts	High ability to track spread based upon movement of infected persons or contacts	Potential ability to track spread based upon movement of infected persons or contacts
Interventions to prevent transmission	International travel restrictions/ screening possible but unlikely to prevent pandemic; quarantine unlikely; school closing and limits on public events likely; vaccination of priority groups	Vaccination effective if given within 4 d of infection	International travel restrictions/ screening possible and likely to help prevent outbreaks; quarantine likely; school closing and limits on public events unlikely
Disruption of transportation infrastructure, community services	Widespread, widespread		Widespread, little

Preventive Medicine

Vaccination when available, social distancing, cough etiquette, hand hygiene

Epidemiological Surveillance

Rapid case investigation, contact tracing, and clusters containment
Quick reporting of suspected cases by affected countries

Clinical Medicine

Delivery of Health Services

Passive case finding but use of influenza clinics and fever hospitals

Standardized Case Management

<u>Case definitions</u>
<u>Treatment protocols</u>
technical expertise in case management including rational use of antiviral treatment and prophylaxis
<u>Essential drugs</u>
monitoring for counterfeit antiviral medications
<u>Referral guidelines</u>
what to do in resource poor settings
<u>Secondary prevention</u>

- health care setting
  - Pt isolation in specific hospital/ward designations
  - private room or cohorting with other flu Pts
  - minimize transport of Pt outside room
  - limit # of HCWs interacting with flu Pt
  - limit # of visitors interacting with flu Pt
  - infection control
    - standard standard precautions with PPE and hand washing
    - contact hand hygiene
    - airborne powered air purifying or N95 respirators, cough suppression
    - droplet N95 respirators
- home setting
  - voluntary Pt isolation in private room
  - minimize transport of Pt outside room
  - limit # of family interacting with flu Pt
  - infection control
    - standard standard precautions with PPE and hand washing

contact hand hygiene
airborne N95 respirators, cough suppression
droplet N95 respirators
voluntary quarantine of contacts of known cases
NB management of contacts (contact tracing, contact monitoring) potentially useful only very early in epidemic
quarantine of close contacts for a complete incubation period potentially useful only very early in epidemic

- all settings—try to decrease potential for infection
  vaccination
  seasonal or post-exposure antiviral chemoprophylaxis
  < susceptibility to infection by 30%
  if infection occurs, < infectiousness by 36%
  if disease occurs, < probability of clinically recognizable Sx by 65%

Epidemic Management

Case definitions may change and become more specific as epidemic evolves
Case management guidelines
Outbreak management protocol

- rapid response teams to investigate case reports
- epidemic investigation kits to mobilize
- specimens to collect
- labs to verify diagnosis and share specimens with peer labs
- contacts to trace and? quarantine
- hotline use and rumor investigation

Secondary prevention

- specific groups of exposed or at risk in the community—most likely to work when there is limited disease transmission in the area, most cases can be traced to a specific contact or setting, and intervention is considered likely to slow the spread of disease
  eg quarantine of groups of people at known common source exposure (airplane, school, workplace, hospital, public gathering; ensure delivery of medical care, food, and social services to persons in quarantine with special attention to vulnerable groups) (useless once there is community-based spread)
  eg containment measures at specific sites or buildings of disease exposure (focused measures to > social distance)
  cancel public events (concerts, sports, movies)
  close buildings (recreational facilities, youth clubs)
  restrict access to certain sites or buildings
- community-wide measures (affecting exposed and non-exposed)—most likely to work where there is moderate to extensive disease transmission in the area, many cases cannot be traced, cases are increasing, and there is delay between Sx onset and case isolation.

infection control measures

ARI etiquette—cover nose/mouth during cough or sneeze, use tissues, wash hands

avoidance of public gatherings by persons at high risk of complications

NB use of masks by well persons is not recommended

"snow" (stay-at-home) days and self-shielding (reverse quarantine) for initial 10 d period of community outbreak—may reduce transmission without explicit activity restrictions

closure of schools, offices, large group gatherings, public transport (pedes more likely to transmit disease than adults)

NB community quarantine (cordon sanitaire)—restriction of travel in and out of an area is unlikely to prevent introduction or spread of disease

- international travel

  NB travel advisories to restrict international travel are generally useless in slowing epidemic spread

  NB health screening for fever and respiratory Sx at ports of entry is also generally useless in slowing epidemic spread

Resource prepositioning, stockpiles, and supply chain management

- facemasks
- PPE
- vaccines, antiviral drugs

Information management

- health workers
- political authorities
- public via awareness campaign and behavior change communication

Contingency planning

- incident/event management system and role designations
- surveillance, investigation, and containment
- vaccines, antivirals
- provision of essential services (lifelines, health care, and emergency response)
- culturally appropriate corpse management

Avian Influenza

Poultry Cases

- Biosecurity
- Cull
- Disposal
- Disinfection
- Control movement
- Quarantine
- Count (surveillance around affected flocks)
- Ring vaccination

Overall approach

primary prevention: animal vaccination (prevents viral reassortment)

cases: biosecurity (of premises), cull, disposal (of carcasses), disinfection (of premises)

contacts: quarantine, control movement, count (surveillance), ring vaccination

Human Cases

- Health Care—infection control (PPE)
- Control movement
- Quarantine
- Count (surveillance)
- Vaccines
- Antiviral drugs

Overall approach

primary prevention: animal vaccination (prevents viral reassortment)

cases: isolation, infection control, antiviral therapy

contacts: quarantine, infection control, count (surveillance), vaccination, antivirals with chemoprophylaxis for high risk persons

NB: travel screening & restrictions, quarantine, and school cancellation are not effective measures.

References

1. World Health Organization and Centers for Disease Control and Prevention. History and epidemiology of global smallpox eradication. In: Smallpox: Disease, Prevention, and Intervention training course, undated. Available from: https://emergency.cdc.gov/agent/smallpox/training/overview/pdf/eradicationhistory.pdf .
2. US Department of Health and Human Services. Pandemic influenza preparedness and response plan draft. Annex 12, p 8–11. August 2004. Available from: US Department of Health and Human Services, Washington, DC.

MALARIA

Pathogen Vectors

Table 7.6.5
Mosquito Biology [1]

Vector group	Species	Breeding sites	Resting sites	Transmission activity	Blood source	Diseases
Anophelines	*Anopheles*	Natural pools of unpolluted water	Indoor/ outdoor	Evening and night	Humans and animals	Malaria, filariasis arboviruses
Culicines	*Aedes*	Water containers (tires), pools of stagnant water	Indoor/ outdoor	Day	Humans and animals	Filariasis, YF, DF
	Culex	Organically polluted water (sewers), natural pools of unpolluted water	Indoor/ outdoor	Day and night	Humans and animals	Filariasis, viral encephalitis
	Mansonia	Unpolluted water with plants	Indoor/ outdoor	Day and night	Humans and animals	Filariasis

Source: M Connolly (ed) in *Communicable disease control in emergencies—a field manual* © 2005. Used with permission of the World Health Organization.

Anopheles vector biology
- egg becomes adult mosquito in 9 d
- adult mosquito becomes infective in 12 d after bite on infected host
- susceptible human host becomes infective in 9 d after bite from infected mosquito
- :. earliest human clinical disease in 30 d after eggs are laid

Preventive Medicine

Health messages
Follow the 4-D rule:
- **d**usk and **d**awn stay indoors as much as possible with window screens in good repair
- **d**ress in light colored long sleeve shirts and long pants when outside

DEET (N,N-diethyl-M-toluamide) based mosquito repellants
drain any standing water from the area (flower pots, old tires, clogged rain gutters, etc); flush troughs, birdbaths, wading pools, etc every 3 days

Insecticides

10% DDT, 1% malathion, 1% permethrin
insecticide treated nets (ITNs) (esp long-lasting nets with duration of 3–5 years)
indoor residual spraying (IRS) (esp within 2 weeks of high transmission season; more effective in Asia than Africa; not appropriate for dengue)

deterrence:	# mosquitoes which don't enter room
repellence:	# mosquitoes which enter then leave room
bite inhibition:	# mosquitoes which enter room but don't bite
direct knock down:	# mosquitoes which are knocked down, but still live
direct death:	# mosquitoes killed

NB aerial spraying & outdoor spraying (fogging) are not especially useful in malaria
deterrence & repellence effectiveness is species-specific (eg aedes > anopheles > culex)
coils work by knockdown effect, not bite inhibition

Larvicides

organophosphate (Temephos—safe for drinking water)
Bacillus thuringiensis israelensis (bacterial toxin)
Mesocyclops copepods (used in Vietnam in village water tanks)
larvivorous fish (used in China in domestic water tanks)

Insect repellents (useful for individuals who can afford it but not as public health intervention)

DEET

Chemoprophylaxis

seasonal malaria chemoprophylaxis (SMC)
international staff travelling to endemic areas
intermittent preventive treatment (IPT) for pregnant women in endemic areas where continuous chemoprophylaxis is not feasible

Generally, control programs rely upon:

3 major components—ITN, IPT, and prompt clinical treatment
2 ancillary components—IRS, environmental clean-up of breeding sites

Epidemiological Surveillance

Geographic reconnaissance

mapping of target area before spraying
mapping of homes for IRS

Entomological survey

night mosquito survey
mosquitoes trapped/hr (calculation of man-biting rate)
species identification
mosquito dissection (F only) to determine parity; % parity inversely related to spraying effectiveness

Malariometric survey
prevalence in sample of 100 persons
spleen rate in sample of 100 persons
slide positivity rate (ratio of # confirmed cases/# clinically suspected cases)
proportion of fever caused by malaria (# fever cases with confirmed parasitemia/# total fevers)

Malaria mortality (# malaria deaths/10,000 p/d for given area)
Case fatality rate in all malaria cases
Case fatality rate in severe malaria cases
Proportional mortality (# malaria deaths/# total deaths)
Malaria incidence rate

Clinical Medicine

Delivery of Health Services

Active case finding through CHWs

Standardized Case Management

Case definition
Pt with F or history of F associated with Sx such as N, V, D, headache, back pain, chills, myalgia, where other infectious diseases have been clinically excluded

Rapid (point of care) diagnostic testing (RDT)
Treatment protocols per local health authorities
Essential drugs
Referral guidelines
Secondary prevention
community education
health messages—printed, loudspeaker, broadcast, community groups
community understands transmission and prevention measures

Epidemic Management

Outbreak management protocol
Secondary prevention
Resource prepositioning (stockpiles & supply chain management)

indoor residual spraying (IRS) (within 2 weeks of epidemic)
mass fever treatment (MFT) (active case finding & fever treatment with antimalarials)
mass drug administration (MDA) (cover 80% of population within 2 weeks)

Information management
Contingency planning

Reference

1. Connolly M (ed). *Communicable disease control in emergencies—a field manual.* Geneva: World Health Organization, 2005.

MEASLES

Preventive Medicine

EPI
Subnational immunization days
Measles immunization of contacts of confirmed case if contacts have <2 doses of vaccine

Epidemiological Surveillance

Surveillance definition becomes clinical once outbreak is lab-confirmed

Clinical Medicine

Delivery of Health Services

Active case finding through CHWs

Standardized Case Management

Case definition
- An illness characterized by all of the following clinical features: a generalized rash lasting greater than or equal to 3 d (exanthems generally without symmetry or pruritis); $T \geq 38.3$ °C (101 °F); cough, or coryza, or conjunctivitis

Treatment protocols emphasizing supportive care and treatment of complications
- Vitamin A

Table 7.6.6 Vitamin A Treatment Schedules in Infant/Child Deficiency States

Age	Initial Dose	Next Day Dose
0–6 months	50,000 IU	50,000 IU
6–11 months	100,000 IU	100,000 IU
1+ years	200,000 IU	200,000 IU

Essential drugs
Referral guidelines
Secondary prevention
- community education
  - health messages—printed, loudspeaker, broadcast, community groups
  - community understands measles transmission and prevention measures

Epidemic Management

Identify cause of the outbreak
Undertake vaccination campaign
Strengthen routine immunization and surveillance

Table 7.6.7
Population Vaccination Status and Contributing Causes

Vaccination Status and Patient Age	Probable Cause
> 50% cases U5 & unvaccinated	low coverage
> 50% cases U5 & vaccinated	not measles, or vaccine ineffective
> 50% cases O5 in high coverage area	disease shift to older age group
high % of cases in infants	low routine coverage

MENINGITIS

Pathogens and Epidemiology

Meningitis is a disease with significant mortality. Meningococcus (*Neisseria meningitides*) is renown for its rapid onset, rapid progression (death sometimes within hours), and high mortality (50% untreated).

There are 13 serogroups of *Neisseria meningitides* but only 6 (A, B, C, W, X, Y) are known to cause epidemics.

The bacteria spread from person to person via respiratory and nasal secretions. Kissing, sharing eating and drinking utensils, cigarettes, coughing, and sneezing are recognized methods of transmission. Close contacts over a period of time, as between household or dormitory residents, are most commonly affected. Population movements (eg pilgrimages, displacement, military recruitment), poor living conditions, and overcrowding are epidemic risk factors.

Large, recurring epidemics of meningitis occur in the "meningitis belt" of sub-Saharan Africa where over 430 million people live. This belt encompasses 26 countries from Senegal in the west to Ethiopia in the east and as far south as Tanzania and the Democratic Republic of Congo. Subsaharan Arica has epidemic seasonality. Dry seasons and droughts favor epidemics. Rains stop them. Large regional epidemics, as well as epidemics in displaced populations and refugee camps, have mainly been due to meningococcus serogroup A. Since 2010, extensive use of meningococcal type A conjugate vaccine in the meningitis belt has reduced the incidence and case load of type A epidemics by nearly 60%. In 2016, the most common lab confirmed meningitis isolate was *Streptococcus pneumoniae.*

In non-epidemic settings, *Neisseria.meningitidis*, *Streptococcus pneumoniae*, and *Haemophilus influenzae* account for 80% of all cases of bacterial meningitis. Prior to the availability of conjugate vaccines, *H. influenza* type b (Hib) was the most common cause of childhood bacterial meningitis outside of epidemics. Where Hib vaccines are in the routine infant immunization schedule, Hib meningitis has nearly disappeared.

Preventive Medicine

Polysaccharide vaccines are available with 2 serotypes (A and C), 3 serotypes (A, C, and W) or 4 serotypes (A, C, W, and Y). Duration of immunity is approximately 3 years.

Meningococcal protein conjugate vaccines confer longer immunity but at higher cost than polysaccharide vaccines. Monovalent conjugate vaccine against group C dates from 1999, and tetravalent (A, C, W, and Y) conjugate vaccine dates from 2005. Group B vaccine made from 4 bacterial proteins has been licensed since 2014 but is not readily available.

Meningococcal vaccines have a very low incidence of side effects.

Epidemiological Surveillance

Regular disease surveillance is necessary to detect outbreaks. The epidemic threshold is 10 suspected cases/ 100,000 population in any given week. Two suspected cases of meningitis in the same settlement should trigger an outbreak investigation.

Nasopharyngeal carriage rates do not predict epidemics.

Clinical Medicine

80–85% of meningococcal disease presents with meningitis. 80% of cases occur in patients <30 y/o. Peak incidence in meningitis belt is ages 5–10 yrs. Diagnosis is straightforward when patient presents with signs of meningitis—fever, headache, vomiting, changes in mental status. However, most patients have non-specific illness 1–3 days before onset of meningitis. CFR of untreated meningococcal meningitis can be 50%. CFR of properly treated meningococcal meningitis is <1%.

15–20% of meningococcal disease presents with septicemia unaccompanied by meningitis or other focal features. It is a dramatic illness which affects previously healthy children and young adults. It presents with acute fever leading to purpura fulminans (hemorrhagic or purpuric rash), shock, and Waterhouse-Friderichsen syndrome (acute adrenal failure). Etiologic diagnosis can be easily missed. CFR of meningococcal septicemia is 50% and may be 25% even with proper treatment.

Diagnosis may be confirmed by agglutination tests, polymerase chain reaction, culture and sensitivity testing of spinal fluid and blood. In many situations, these tests are not available. Throat swabs may be helpful on occasions. **Do not delay treatment for tests or test results. Minutes count. It is more important to have a live patient without a confirmed diagnosis than a dead one with a diagnosis**.

Differential diagnosis in a tropical patient with fever and altered mental status, but without purpura or shock, includes cerebral malaria. Co-infection may occur.

Standardized case management of bacterial meningitis in developed countries involves 7–10 days of parenteral antibiotic therapy. Drug of choice in adults and older children is ceftriaxone which also rapidly eliminates the carrier state. Alternate drugs include ampicillin and benzylpenicillin which do not eliminate the carrier state. In developing countries, 4 days of parenteral antibiotic therapy are empirically shown to be effective. In large epidemics in resource-poor settings, a single IM dose of chloramphenicol in oil is the drug of choice. For patients who do not improve in 48 hours, a repeat dose may be given.

Viral meningitis is rarely serious and requires only supportive care, Recovery is usually complete.

Patient isolation and disinfection of the room, clothing, or bedding are not necessary. Respiratory precautions are advised particularly early in the course of treatment.

Chemoprophylaxis of contacts is available in some settings but rarely in the disaster setting. Vigilance and education of close contacts is mandatory.

Epidemic Management

Epidemic preparedness and early detection of outbreaks are key.

Vaccines against *N. meningitides* serogroups A, C, Y and W135 are very effective in controlling epidemics. In epidemic settings, children 2–10 are the priority target with serogroups A and C typically the priority antigens. Rapid mass vaccination campaigns can contain outbreaks in 2–3 weeks. For immunocompetent patients over 2 years, vaccine efficacy rate is 90% one week after injection. However, duration of immunity may be as little as 2 years in younger children. In some countries, vaccine may also be used with close contacts of sporadic disease cases to prevent secondary cases.

Chemoprophylaxis of contacts is not recommended in epidemics, but community education and ready access to health care are essential.

VIRAL HEMORRHAGIC FEVER

Preventive Medicine [1]

Source control/reduction/elimination
- Undertake quarantine and culling of sick reservoir animals and known disease carrier species.
- Avoid unnecessary contact with or consumption of dead reservoir animals or known disease carrier species.
- Avoid unnecessary contact with suspected reservoir animals and known disease carrier species (eg primates).
- Avoid direct or close contact with symptomatic patients.
- Establish appropriate communicable disease controls for burial of the dead.

Administrative controls (improve people's work practices)

Environmental and engineering controls (isolate people from the hazard)
- Avoid needle stick exposure to blood specimens thru automated machine handling.

PPE (protect people with PPE)
- Use standard precautions—gloves, masks, and protective clothing—if handling infected animals or patients.
- Wash hands after visiting sick patients.

Epidemiological Surveillance

Active surveillance and contact tracing (enhanced surveillance) through community-based mobile teams

Clinical Medicine [2]

Delivery of Health Services

Active case finding (screening and triage) and contact tracing
Dedicated isolation facility
Food provision to isolated patients so they are not dependent on family

Standardized Case Management

Case definition
Treatment protocols emphasizing supportive care and treatment of complications
Essential drugs
Referral guidelines
Secondary prevention
- barrier nursing strictly enforced
- family and community education

Epidemic Management

Ministerial task force to address policy
Local health authority task force to address procedures
National level task forces to comprise

- Response unit
  - epidemiology (case finding, contact tracing, monitoring, surveillance)
  - facilities preparation (build beds)
  - case management
  - laboratory
  - infection prevention and control (IPC) (including safe burial)
  - social mobilization, communication
  - training
- Support unit (manage resources)
  - program & HR planning (16 positions)
  - staffing model
    1. social/medical/cultural anthropologist
    2. social mobilization/community engagement specialist
    3. social mobilization coordinator at national level
    4. epidemiologist
    5. IPC specialist
    6. PH advisor
    7. subnational field coordinator
    8. VHF lab specialist
    9. case management specialist
    10. EMTs
    11. occupational health and safety specialist
    12. logistics
    13. exit screening
    14. data management
    15. health communications
    16. finance
- Research unit
  - new therapeutics
  - new tests
  - clinical trials
  - analytic epi and modelling
- Long term measures
  - health systems recovery

Outbreak management in the field focuses on

- alert verification
- disease surveillance (not relying exclusively or even largely on health facility reporting)
- burial <48 hrs after death
- spot checking of contact tracing effectiveness (< 5 is inadequate; 25–50 is reasonable; 75 is not extreme)

- door-to-door community education campaigns
- quarantine sustainment at HH level

  NB it's difficult to separate ebola from non-ebola fevers at onset, so holding centers can amplify transmission

Secondary prevention

Resource prepositioning (stockpiles & supply chain management)

Information management—refute travel and trade restrictions

Community education and social mobilization

- health messages—printed, loudspeaker, broadcast, community groups
- community understands disease transmission and prevention measures

Contingency planning

References

1. World Health Organization. Ebola: technical guidance documents for medical staff. Available from: https://www.who.int/csr/disease/ebola/protective-measures-staff/en/. Accessed January 2019.
2. World Health Organization. Manual for the care and management of patients in ebola care units/community care centers—interim emergency guidance. WHO/EVD/Manual/ECU/15.1. Geneva: World Health Organization; January 2015. Available from: https://www.who.int/csr/resources/publications/ebola/ebola-preparedness-checklist/en/. Accessed January 2018.

Document 7.7
DIAGNOSTIC LABORATORY

Glossary

Ab	antibody
AFB	acid-fast bacilli
Ag	antigen
C&S	culture and antibiotic sensitivity
CIE	counterimmunoelectrophoresis
COTS	Cholera Outbreak Training and Shigellosis Program (training program developed at ICDDR)
CSF	cerebrospinal fluid
ELISA	enzyme-linked immunosorbent assay
d	day
HAI	hemagglutination inhibition
IgG, IgM	immunoglobulin G, M
O&P	ova and parasite (stool slide examination)
PCR	polymerase chain reaction
Pt	patient
RDT	rapid diagnostic test
TB	tuberculosis

Lab Purposes

- Confirm syndromic or clinical diagnosis
  - Identify treatment options
  - Identify control measures
- Characterize the agent (serotype, biotype, antibiogram, etc.)
  - Evaluate potential effectiveness of treatment
  - Monitor the spread of a particular clone or subtype
- Detect an outbreak and confirm its end

Key Questions on Lab (WHO [1])

1. Is a laboratory available?
2. What tests does it perform?
3. Is there transport to and from the laboratory?
4. Who prepares transport media?
5. Who provides specimen collection material and supplies?
6. How can these supplies be obtained?
7. Who provides cool packs, transport boxes, car, driver …?
8. What forms/information must be sent with the specimens?
9. What epidemiological information must accompany test results?
10. How does the epidemiologist obtain results?

If a lab is not available, then you need a sampling strategy that addresses specimen acquisition, preparation, and transportation in compliance with international regulations on the transport of infectious substances.

Table 7.7.1
Indications, Laboratory Tests, and Expected Availability

Cases	Lab Tests	PHC Clinic	Confirmation Laboratory
Watery diarrhea—dehydrating (suspected cholera)	• Fine microscopy for motility on wet prep, O&P • Gram's stain • Stool C&S • Toxin or polysaccharide (RDT)	• + • + • +/– • ?	• District lab • District lab • District lab • District lab
Diarrhea with blood (shigella, salmonella, amoeba)	• Fine microscopy for O&P • Stool C&S	• + • +/–	• District lab • District lab
Acute respiratory infection	• Strep screen, throat C&S • Microscopy with Ziehl-Neelsen stain for AFB	• + • +	• District lab • District lab
Acute febrile illness (suspected malaria)	• Microscopy with Giemsa stain • Ag detection (RDT)	• + • +	• District lab • District lab
Acute febrile illness (suspected typhoid)	• Blood culture • Serology (ELISA, RDT)	• – • –	• District lab • District lab
Meningitis (suspected meningococcus)	• CSF microscopy with Gram's stain • CSF C&S • CSF PCR	• + • – • –	• District lab • District lab • District lab
Acute jaundice syndrome (suspected viral hepatitis)	• Serology	• –	• District lab
Acute flaccid paralysis (suspected poliomyelitis)	• Virus isolation (cell culture from stool specimens)	• –	• Reference lab
Measles	• Serology (IgM)	None—clinical Dx	• District lab
Neonatal tetanus	None—clinical Dx	None—clinical Dx	None—clinical Dx

Cases	Lab Tests	PHC Clinic	Confirmation Laboratory
Acute febrile illness (suspected influenza)	• Ag detection (RDT—Types A, B) • PCR	• ? • –	• District lab • District lab
Acute febrile illness (suspected dengue fever)	• Ab detection (RDT) immunochromatography • Serology (IgM of paired sera) • PCR	• – • – • –	• District lab • District lab • Reference lab
Leptospirosis	• Ab detection (RDT) • Serology (ELISA)	• – • –	• Reference lab • Reference lab
Typhus	• Serology	• –	• Reference lab

Direct techniques

1. microscopy (direct visualization)
2. culture (isolation)
3. immunological Ag techniques—immunohistochemistry, immunochromatography
   molecular Ag techniques—DNA or RNA PCR, antigen capture

Indirect serological (Ab) techniques

1. bacterial agglutination
2. hemagglutination inhibition assay
3. ELISA for IgM, IgG
4. microneutralization assay

NB non-specific response from some organisms
little or no response in host immunosuppression
delays in serological response oblige testing of early and late sera

Table 7.7.2
Specimen Handling (adapted from WHO [1])

Issue	Clinical and lab details			
When to sample?	Early stages of infection, during peaks of fever, and before ABX.			
	• Acute diarrhea • Acute flaccid paralysis	• Meningitis	• Fevers • Icterus • Measles	• Misc
What to sample?	• Stool	• Cerebrospinal fluid	• Whole blood	• Sputum for TB • Urine for schisto, lepto • Bubo aspirate for plague
How many samples and how often to sample?	• 10–20 samples (different Pts) initially to confirm outbreak • 10–20 samples each month to verify strain and drug susceptibility (systematic random sampling with skip interval of monthly total visits/sample size) • 10–20 samples (different Pts) after epidemic to confirm resolution (COTS avoids this as cholera or shigella usually causes <5% of all diarrhea outside of epidemic)	• Similar to stool protocol but half the number	• 10 samples initially, but strategy may vary with disease • Paired samples for serology—early and after 7–14 d	

Biosafety while sampling?	• Protect yourself (universal precautions, personal protective equipment as needed) • Protect the Pt (disinfect, use single use materials) • Protect the environment (waste disposal, triple package the specimen)			
How to sample?	• Collect liquid stool in leak-proof container • Use forceps to immerse swab or filter paper dots in liquid stool • Place in specimen container with a few drops of sterile saline • For bloody stool, sample several areas of specimen including blood, mucous, or tissue	• Lumbar puncture in usual way	• Venipuncture in usual way	
How to prepare the sample?	• Cary Blair* • Trans Isolate (cost high) • Alcaline peptone water (if <6 h before plating) • saline solution	• Trans Isolate+	• Whole blood for CBC, microscopy (purple cap—EDTA tube) • Serum for serology (red cap—no additive; orange cap—gel separator) • Whole blood for blood culture (biphasic culture bottle—10% blood to media ratio) obtain before starting ABX • Blood smear for malaria microscopy	

(continued)

Table 7.7.2 (continued)

Issue	Clinical and lab details			
How to preserve and send the sample?	• Refrigerate if possible (4 °C) or cool packs	• Incubate Trans Isolate for culture (25–37 °C) • Refrigerate other vials for cytology, chemistry (4 °C)	• Incubate blood culture (25–37 °C) • Refrigerate sera (4–8 °C) • Ambient temp for smears	• Refrigerate specimen (4 °C)
	Triple package in appropriate packaging (eg local official container or consistent with international regulation 650) 1. Leak-proof specimen container wrapped with enough absorbent material to absorb the entire content of the 1st container 2. Leak-proof secondary container usually plastic or metal 3. Outer shipping container whose smallest dimension is 10 mm Diagnostic specimens use IATA packing instruction 650 without biohazard label. Infectious materials use IATA packing instruction 602 with biohazard label.			
What to send with the sample?	Lab request form with: • Sender's name and contact info • Patient name, age, sex • Sample date, time • Suspected clinical diagnosis with main signs and symptoms • Sample macroscopic description • Context—outbreak confirmation, ongoing verification, outbreak end, etc • Epidemiological or demographic data			
Where to send the sample?	• Reference lab • Contact person			
What and when to expect results?				

Source: World Health Organization. Highlights of specimen collection in emergency situations. Undated. Used with permission of WHO.

* Semi-solid transport medium, easy to use
Place swab with sample in medium to immerse tip of swab. Break off wooden swab handle. Cap tightly.
Use with stool and other samples containing non-fragile bacterial pathogens.
Inexpensive medium. Long shelf life after preparation (about 1 year at 25° C). Can be prepared in advance and pre-positioned at peripheral levels.

\+ Biphasic transport medium with agar and broth
Pre-warm medium to 25–37° C before inoculation. Place 1 cc of specimen in sterile medium for culture. Immediately incubate or hold at 25–37° C. Ventilate bottle if >4 days to lab.
Place 1 cc of specimen in another sterile vial for cytology, chemistry, and CIE. Refrigerate.
More expensive medium.

Reference

1. World Health Organization Department of Communicable Disease Surveillance and Response. Highlights of specimen collection in emergency situations. Undated. Available from: WHO Laboratory and Epidemiology Capacity Strengthening Office in Lyon, France, and http://www.who.int/hac/techguidance/training/highlights%20of%20specimen%20collection_en.pdf. Accessed June 9, 2017.

Document 7.8
ACRONYMS

ABC	abstain until marriage, be faithful, use condoms
ACAPS	Assessment Capacities Project
ACT	artemisinin-based combination therapy
ADB	Asian Development Bank
AfDB	African Development Bank Group
AFRO	Africa Regional Office (WHO)
AI	avian influenza
AIDS	acquired immune deficiency syndrome
AKF	Aga Khan Foundation
ALDAC	all diplomatic and consular posts (USG)
ALNAP	Active Learning Network for Accountability and Performance (ODI)
AMB E&P	Ambassador Extraordinary and Plenipotentiary
AMRO	Americas Regional Office (WHO)
APS	annual program statement (USAID\OFDA statement of funding opportunities for NGOs)
APW	agreement for the performance of work (WHO contractual work agreement)
ARI	acute respiratory infection
ART	antiretroviral therapy
AU	African Union
BCC	behavior change communication
BCP	business continuity planning
BIC	basic internet communications
BMS	breast milk substitute
BSL	biosafety security level
BWI	Bretton Woods Institutions (World Bank and International Monetary Fund)
CA	cooperative agreement
CAP	consolidated appeals process (supplanted in 2013 by the humanitarian programme cycle; led by OCHA)
CBJ	Congressional budget justification
CBO	community-based organization
CBPF	country-based pooled funds (amalgamation of Emergency Response Funds and Common Humanitarian Funds administered by OCHA)
CBRNE	chemical, biological, radiological, nuclear, or explosive
CCCM	camp coordination and camp management
CCS	country cooperation strategy (WHO)
CCTV	closed-circuit television
CD	communicable diseases
CDC	communicable disease control; Centers for Disease Control and Prevention (US)

CE	complex emergency
CERF	Central Emergency Response Fund (administered by OCHA)
CFE	Contingency Fund for Emergencies (WHO)
CHW	community health worker
CLA	cluster lead agency
CMAM	community-based management of acute malnutrition
CMOC	civil-military operations center
CMR	crude mortality rate
CO	country office (WHO)
COD	common operational dataset
CoDel	Congressional Delegation
COG	continuity of government
CONOPS	concept of operations
CoOp	continuity of operations
COP	common operating picture
CPA	comprehensive peace agreement
CRED	Center for Research on the Epidemiology of Disasters (Belgium)
CSP	certified safety professional
CSW	commercial sex worker
CTC	community therapeutic care (of malnutrition)
CTO	cognizant technical officer
CTP	cash transfer program
DA	development assistance—US Congress appropriated funds with tight reporting requirements
DANIDA	Danish International Development Agency
DART	Disaster Assistance Response Team (USAID)
DCHA	Bureau for Democracy, Conflict, and Humanitarian Assistance (USAID)
DDR(P)	disarmament, demobilization, and reintegration program
DDRR(P)	disarmament, demobilization, rehabilitation, and reintegration program
DDRRR(P)	disarmament, demobilization, repatriation, resettlement, and reintegration program
DFID	Department for International Development (UK)
DHN	digital humanitarian network
DHO	District Health Office
DMAT	Disaster Medical Assistance Team (US)
DM/HA	disaster management and humanitarian assistance
DMORT	Disaster Mortuary Operational Response Team
DO	designated official (UN)
DOD	Department of Defense (US)
DOS	Department of State (US)
DOTS	direct observed therapy short-course (used for TB)
DRM	disaster risk management

DRR	disaster risk reduction
DS	diplomatic security
DTM	displacement tracking matrix
ECHO	European Community Humanitarian Office (European Commission Directorate General for Humanitarian Aid and Civil Protection which uses ECHO acronym)
EDG	Emergency Directors' Group
EHK	emergency health kit
EIA	environmental impact assessment
EMRO	Eastern Mediterranean Regional Office (WHO)
EMS	Emergency Medical Services
EMT	Emergency Medical Team
EOC	Emergency Operations Center
EOD	explosive ordnance disposal
EPI	Expanded Programme on Immunization
ERC	Emergency Relief Coordinator (UN)
ERF	Emergency Response Framework (WHO)
ERT	Emergency Response Team (WHO)
ESF	emergency school feeding
EST	Emergency Support Team (WHO)
ETS	Emergency telecommunications sector
EU	European Union
EURO	European Regional Office (WHO)
EWAR, EWS	early warning system
EWARN	Early Warning Alert and Response Network
FACT	Field Assessment Coordination Team (IFRC)
FAO	Food and Agriculture Organization (UN)
FCV	fragility, conflict, and violence
FEMA	Federal Emergency Management Agency (US)
FETP	Field Epidemiology Training Program
FEWS	Famine Early Warning Systems
FEWS NET	Famine Early Warning Systems Network
FFA	food assistance for assets (formerly food for work)
FFP	Food for Peace (USAID\DCHA office)
FOG	*Field Operations Guide* (OFDA)
FSN	foreign service national
FSO	field security officer
FTS	Financial Tracking Service (OCHA)
FY	fiscal year
G 7	group of 7 countries
G 20	group of 20 countries
G 77	group of 77 countries
GAM	global acute malnutrition (moderate + severe acute malnutrition)
GBV	gender-based violence
GDACS	Global Disaster Alert and Coordination System
GDP	gross domestic product

GEMT	Global Emergency Management Team (WHO)
GFATM	Global Fund to Fight AIDS, Tuberculosis and Malaria
GFD	general food distribution
GFDRR	Global Facility for Disaster Reduction and Recovery (WB)
GHC	Global Health Cluster
GHD	good humanitarian donorship (initiated by DFID)
GHSA	Global Health Security Agenda
GIC	Global Impact Charities (consortium of faith-based organizations involved in HA)
GIEWS	Global Information and Early Warning System (FAO)
GIS	geographic information system
GNP	gross national product
GO	governmental organization
GOARN	Global Outbreak Alert and Response Network
GPN	global private network
GTZ	German Technical Cooperation
HA	humanitarian assistance
HAART	highly active anti-retroviral treatment
HAZMAT	hazardous materials
HBP	Health as a Bridge for Peace (WHO headquarters program initiative, now discontinued)
HC	Humanitarian Coordinator (IASC)
HCC	Health Cluster Coordinator
HCT	Humanitarian Country Team
HCW	health care worker
HDR	humanitarian daily ration
HELP	Health Emergencies in Large Populations (ICRC training course)
HEPA	high efficiency particulate aspirator (air filter)
HeRAMS	Health Resources Availability and Mapping System
HEWS	Humanitarian Early Warning System
HH	household
HHA	humanitarian health assistance
HHS	Department of Health and Human Services (US)
HIC	Humanitarian Information Centre (OCHA)
HIS	health information system
HIU	Humanitarian Information Unit (US DOS)
HIV	human immunodeficiency virus
HNO	humanitarian needs overview
HOA	Head of Agency
HPAI	highly pathogenic avian influenza
HPC	humanitarian programme cycle
HPF	humanitarian pooled fund
HRP	humanitarian response plan (akin to SRP)
HWCO	Head of WHO Country Office

IAHE	interagency humanitarian evaluation (IASC process, triggered by L3 declaration, to be done within 12 m of declaration)
IAP	incident action plan
IASC	Interagency Standing Committee
IATA	International Air Transport Association
IBRD	International Bank for Reconstruction and Development (World Bank)
ICC	International Criminal Court
ICCG	Intercluster Coordination Group
ICDDR	International Centre for Diarrhoeal Disease Research, Bangladesh
ICMH	International Centre for Migration and Health
ICRC	International Committee of the Red Cross
ICS	Incident Command System
ID	infectious disease
IDA	International Development Association
IDFA	international disaster and famine account—US Congress appropriated funds which have no Congressional Note reporting requirements (see DA)
IDLH	immediately dangerous to life and health
IDP	internally displaced person
IDSR	Integrated Disease Surveillance and Response (AFRO initiative expanded to other regions)
IDU	injection drug user
IEC	information, education, and communication materials
IED	improvised explosive device
IEIP	International Emerging Infections Programs—foreign centers of excellence working in partnership with domestic MOH and US CDC which train local scientists, provide diagnostic and epi resources in outbreaks, and undertake regional disease control activities
IFRC	International Federation of Red Cross and Red Crescent Societies
IGS	income generating scheme
IHL	international humanitarian law
IHR	International Health Regulations
IHRL	international human rights law
ILI	influenza-like illness
IMAI	Integrated Management of Adult Illness (WHO initiative)
IMCI	Integrated Management of Childhood Illness (WHO initiative)
IMF	International Monetary Fund
IMS	incident management system
INSARAG	International Search and Rescue Advisory Group

IO	international organization
IOM	International Organization for Migration
IPC	Integrated Food Security Phase Classification
IRA	initial rapid assessment
IRC	International Rescue Committee
IRIN	Integrated Regional Information Network (OCHA)
ISDR	International Strategy for Disaster Reduction
ITN	insecticide treated nets
ITPS	insecticide treated plastic sheeting
ITWL	insecticide treated wall lining
IYCFE	infant and young child feeding in emergencies
JICA	Japan International Cooperation Agency
L3	level 3 (system-wide) emergency (supplanted by scale-up process)
LOU	letter of understanding
M&E	monitoring and evaluation
MCH	maternal and child health
MCI	mass casualty incident
MDGs	millennium development goals (supplanted by sustainable development goals)
MDM	Médecins du Monde
MDRO	Mission Disaster Relief Officer (USAID)
MEAL	monitoring, evaluation, accountability, and learning
MEB	minimum expenditure basket
MEDS	minimum essential datasets
MICS	multiple indicator cluster survey
MIRA	multi-cluster initial rapid assessment
MIS	management information system
MISP	minimum initial service package (used in reproductive health)
MOH	Ministry of Health
MOSS	minimum operating security standards (UNDSS)
MOU	memorandum of understanding
MSF	Médecins sans Frontières
MUAC	mid-upper arm circumference
NAF	needs analysis framework
NATO	North Atlantic Treaty Organization
NDMA	National Disaster Management Agency
NDMS	National Disaster Medical System (US)
NFI	non-food item (emergency relief supplies)
NGO	non-governmental organization
NIC	National Influenza Center
NICS	nutritional information in crisis situations
NID	national immunization day
NIH	National Institutes of Health (US)
NIMA	National Imagery and Mapping Agency (US)
NRC	Norwegian Refugee Council

NRF	National Response Framework (US)
NSS	National Security Staff (US)
NWOW	new way of working
NZODA	New Zealand Official Development Assistance
OCHA	Office for the Coordination of Humanitarian Affairs (UN)
ODI	Overseas Development Institute (UK)
OECD	Organization for Economic Cooperation and Development
OFDA	Office of US Foreign Disaster Assistance (USAID)
OHCHR	Office of the High Commissioner for Human Rights (UN)
OHCT	Operational Humanitarian Country Team (subnational level)
OIE	Office International des Epizooties (World Organization for Animal Health)
OPD	outpatient department
OPR	operational peer review (IASC process, triggered by L3 declaration, to be done within 90 d of declaration)
ORS	oral rehydration salts/solution
OSCE	Office for Security and Cooperation in Europe
OSOCC	On-Site Operations Coordination Center (UN)
OVC	orphans and vulnerable children
PAHO	Pan-American Health Organization (precursor to and functionally synonymous with AMRO)
PCC	Policy Coordination Committee of the NSC
PDD	Presidential Decision Directive
PDNA	post-disaster needs assessment
PEF	Pandemic Emergency Financing Facility (WB)
PEP	post-exposure prophylaxis
PEPFAR	President's Emergency Plan for AIDS Relief (US)
PHC	primary health care
PHEIC	public health event of international concern (IHR)
PHO	Provincial Health Office
PIO	public international organization
PKO	peace-keeping organization
PLWHA	person living with HIV/AIDS
PMTCT	prevention of mother-to-child transmission
PNG	persona non grata
POC	point of contact
POLR	provider of last resort
PPE	personal protective equipment
PPM	parts per million = mg/L (1 ppm = 1 mg/L = .0001% active ingredient)
PPRR	prevention, preparedness, response, and recovery
PRA	participatory rural appraisal (successor to the RRA)

PRRA	participatory rapid rural appraisal
PSC	personal services contractor
PSD	protective security detail
PSF	Pharmaciens Sans Frontières
PVO	private and voluntary organization
R2D	relief to development
R2P	responsibility to protect
R4	repatriation, reintegration, rehabilitation, and reconstruction
R&R	rest and recreation
RBM	Roll Back Malaria (WHO program)
RC	Resident Coordinator (UN)
REA	rapid epidemiological assessment
RFA	request for assistance
RFI	request for information
RFP	request for proposal
RFQ	request for quote
RH	reproductive health
RMO	Regional Medical Officer (US Department of State)
RMT	Response Management Team (USAID)
RNI	recommended nutritional intake (successor to the recommended daily allowance (RDA))
RO	regional office
RRA	rapid rural appraisal; rapid response account (WHO)
RRM	rapid response mechanism
RRT	rapid response team
RSO	Regional Security Officer (US Department of State)
SAG	strategic advisory group
SAR	search and rescue
SARS	severe acute respiratory syndrome
SBU	sensitive but unclassified
SC	Security Council (UN)
SCF	Save the Children Foundation
SCI	secret compartmented information
SDGs	sustainable development goals
SEARO	South-East Asia Regional Office (WHO)
SGBV	sexual and gender-based violence
SHOC	Strategic Health Operations Center (WHO)
SMART	Standardized Monitoring and Assessment of Relief and Transitions
SME	subject matter expert
SMS	Security Management System (UN)
SMT	Security Management Team (UN)
SNS	Strategic National Stockpile (US)
SO	strategic objective (> 5 yrs to achieve)
SOD	sudden onset disaster

SOG	standard operating guideline
SOP	standard operating procedure
SPHC	selective primary health care
SPHERE	project of humanitarian agencies detailing a humanitarian charter and minimum standards
SpO	special objective (< 5 yrs to achieve)
SRP	strategic response plan
SRSG	Special Representative of the Secretary General (UN)
STI	sexually transmitted infection
SUMA	supply management (PAHO/WHO program)
SWAP	sector-wide approach
TAG	Technical Assistance Group (USAID\OFDA)
TB	tuberculosis
TBA	traditional birth attendant
TFC	therapeutic feeding center
TFP	therapeutic feeding program
TOR	terms of reference
TWG	technical working group
UN	United Nations
UNAIDS	Joint United Nations AIDS Programme
UNCT	UN Country Team
UNDAC	UN Disaster Assessment and Coordination team
UNDAF	UN Development Assistance Framework
UNDMT	UN Disaster Management Team
UNDP	UN Development Programme
UNDPKO	UN Department of Peacekeeping Operations
UNDSS	UN Department of Safety and Security
UNEP	UN Environmental Programme
UNFPA	UN Fund for Population Activities
UNGA	UN General Assembly
UNHAS	UN Humanitarian Air Service (WFP)
UNHCHR	UN High Commissioner for Human Rights
UNHCR	UN High Commissioner for Refugees
UNHRD	UN Humanitarian Response Depot
UNICEF	UN Children's Fund
UNJLC	UN Joint Logistics Center
UNPKO	UN Peace-keeping Operations
UNRC	UN Resident Coordinator
UNSE	UN Special Envoy
UNSG	UN Secretary General
UNV	UN volunteer
USAID	US Agency for International Development
USAR	urban search and rescue
USCR	US Committee for Refugees
USD	US dollar
USDA	US Department of Agriculture

USG	Under Secretary General (UN); US Government
USPHS	US Public Health Service
UXO	unexploded ordnance
VAC	Vulnerability Assessment Committee
VAM	vulnerability assessment and mapping (WFP)
VCT	voluntary counseling and testing (HIV)
WASH	water, sanitation, and hygiene
WB	World Bank
WCO	WHO Country Office
WFP	World Food Programme (UN)
WHE	WHO Health Emergencies Programme
WHO	World Health Organization (UN)
WHZ	weight-for-height z score
WMD	weapons of mass destruction
WPRO	Western Pacific Regional Office (WHO)
WR	WHO Representative (replaced by HWCO)
WWWW, 4 W	who does what where when (matrix)

8 Resilience and Reentry

Contents

Overview

This section provides guidance on resilience and reentry. The challenge for the responder is to develop a robust personal resilience strategy before deployment and a reentry strategy before return. Resilience has physical and psychological components. These components can be embedded in a series of "schedules" for activities of daily living in disaster.

This section focuses on 7 dominant schedules.

- Work
- Sleep
- Eating
- Exercise
- Recreation
- Socialization
- Meditation

All these schedules may be difficult to implement in the hyperacute phase of a sudden onset disaster or the exacerbated phase of a complex disaster. Individual schedules may be difficult to sustain over the course of any disaster. Nonetheless, each individual schedule contributes to personal resilience, and its effect can be synergistic—diet fuels exercise, exercise

D. A. Bradt, C. M. Drummond, *Pocket Field Guide for Disaster Health Professionals*,
https://doi.org/10.1007/978-3-030-04801-3_8

contributes to sleep quality, sleep quality contributes to work quality, etc. Moreover, intact schedules among the seven can mitigate the effects of interruption to other schedules.

Reentry can be the hardest part of the mission. Your heightened awareness may be totally out of sync with the priorities and values of the society you reenter. The disconnect can be disturbing. Disaster relief can also have a polarizing effect on people you meet. Recognize that reentry is an issue for all repatriating staff. You are likely to go thru it tired, jet lagged, distracted, irritable, and perhaps intolerant—the antithesis of resilient. Nonetheless, recognize the stakes are high. Collateral damage in a poorly executed reentry can adversely affect yourself, your family, and your friends. Hence, reentry deserves the same attention to detail as deployment.

Document 8.1
RESILIENCE CHECKLIST

A. Preparedness

1. Understand the 7 schedules of resilience—work, sleep, eating, exercise, recreation, socialization, and meditation.
2. Practice techniques to develop mastery over the schedules—particularly for sleep, exercise, and meditation.
3. Understand the 3 step genesis of accidents and injuries—risky conditions, faulty judgment, and unsafe acts.
4. Understand the differences between flameout, burnout, and post-traumatic stress. These stress reactions have vastly different therapeutic implications.
5. Read the experience of your predecessors. *Deep Survival* and *The Gift of Fear* are core content. *Emergency Sex* is to humanitarian assistance what *The House of God* is to academic medicine.
6. Think of rejuvenating activities you can do in the field. Pack items that may assist—list of exercises, adjuncts (eg stretch belts, exercise mat), small musical instrument, DVDs, cards, books.
7. Work out the ABCs of stress management YOU will do in a hyperacute situation.

B. On Mission

1. Remember that team safety and security are the first priorities and may preempt attention to other issues.
2. Rehearse the plans and skills in lethal situation management. Familiarity creates confidence and competence.
3. Establish a buddy system within the team. It is a fundamental strategy in group safety and security, and affirms expectations that reaching out to each other is important.
4. Be aware of other members of your team and how they are faring. Consider task team assignments and periodic socialization to help build esprit de corps and maintain resilience.
5. Bond with people who have mastered the craft. They can change your life, and may even save it.
6. Make new friends among the locals. They are your early warning system. Learn a few key words of the local language.
7. Try to allocate time each day for your resilience activities. Avoid routines in high threat areas, but incorporate resilience activities into your daily schedule even if only for a few minutes.
8. Learn stress management techniques you can do unobtrusively during the day and in your chair. Find time for relaxation activities before sleep. Engage in activities you found relaxing at home.
9. Prioritize your work. Learn to say no to things that are not priority tasks. Focus on the things that only you can do. Delegate tasks as appropriate.

10. When you have little experience with a new situation, learn to ask insightful questions and seek relevant counsel. The practice affirms the mindset that you don't have to have all the answers, but are smart enough to find them. The practice also makes it easier for you to reach out when issues become personal.
11. Impulse control—observing, measuring, and thinking—may be the best initial response to a crisis situation.
12. Beware of sexual contacts and promiscuity. Sex with team members, locals, prostitutes, or beneficiaries has progressive moral hazard and legal consequence. You can end up with HIV, without a job, and in jail.
13. Stay positive and control your thoughts. Negativity is both a poison and an infectious disease.
14. Minimize alcohol and avoid illicit drugs.
15. Learn to tell a joke. Jokes on you are the best.
16. When things are bad, take them 1 day at a time. When things are really bad, take them 5 minutes at a time. Stay alert, control your breathing, think clearly, and act decisively.
17. Talk through bad news with someone you like and trust.
18. Seek beauty in your environment. The stars at night are beautiful even if you are surrounded by death and destruction.
19. Try not to lose your compassion.

Document 8.2
REENTRY CHECKLIST

A. Field Exit

1. A briefing book for your successor takes days to prepare. See Medical Handover Checklist in Section 2. Try to compile it incrementally instead of waiting until your end-of-mission.
2. Try to complete your end-of-mission report in the field. You don't want to bring back homework from the field. Try to get your report in early to colleagues with whom you will debrief.
3. Inform your field counterparts of your upcoming departure, make courtesy rounds with significant decision-makers, and leave them a token of esteem. You may never see them again, but your successor will inherit the relationship.
4. Try to debrief with your successor in the field, your country office, and your headquarters. You will be lucky if you get 2 out of 3.
5. Try to schedule regional R&R before you leave the field. Regional World Heritage Sites are well-worth visiting, and post-disaster hotel rates away from the relief community are never cheaper.

B. Reentry Home

1. Schedule plenty of rest and relaxation on your return. Avoid going straight back to work.
2. Don't over-program your days. You will probably have acute jet lag and chronic sleep debt.
3. Try not to make a significant decision or undertake a life event immediately on your return.
4. Try not to schedule yourself for clinical duties on your return. Admin, teaching, and research duties will generally be less demanding.
5. If you feel sick, seek a primary care provider or travel clinic. If you feel quite ill (high fever, rigor, malaise), seek a hospital emergency department. Do not delay. Tell them where you been been and request a work-up for endemic pathogens—malaria, occult bacteremia, arboviral disease, etc.
6. Don't expect your intimate partner to understand what you did in the field.
7. Don't expect your family and social friends to understand what you did in the field.
8. Don't expect your professional colleagues to understand what you did in the field—unless they are disaster trained, field experienced, and insightful to the craft. Even then, disaster tourism pervades the professional world and masquerades as disaster expertise.

9. Make time for an intimate partner—in a neutral area away from the domestic "real world." Both partners have paid a price for separation. Don't assume you fully understand each other. Give peace a chance.
10. Reach out to your friends, but lower your expectations. Your recent experiences can disconnect you from even your best friends.
11. Reach out to a mentor who knows you well and knows the field. He/she can help you process your experience. Those relationships can be among the most rewarding of your life.
12. Remember the concept of the 7 schedules. Reestablish the habits you found relaxing before your mission.
13. If you experience difficulty with reentry, avoid provocative agents—alcohol and illicit drugs. Seek support from someone you like and trust over a cup of coffee (in decreasing order of helpfulness: someone on your mission > someone who works for the parent organization > someone who has worked in the country of assignment > someone familiar with the region).
14. If you don't find support from the above, seek referral to an expert in adjustment disorders. The management principles are well-worked out, and outcomes from early referral are good.

Epilogue

Disaster health professionals have the privilege of assisting disaster survivors return to marginal self-sufficiency. There are many dedicated health professionals who have fashioned a career in disaster relief. Some careerists have distinguished themselves by advancing selected disaster best practices. A few superbly competent leaders, with inter-disciplinary, inter-agency, and international expertise, have pioneered the modern profession of humanitarian health assistance. They are the masters of the craft.

These masters of the craft are charismatic, observant, innovative, bold, and daring. They see and do things most health professionals cannot. Fortunately, they have identified their keys to mastery—rules of engagement—that enable others to best make their own contribution.

Skip Burkle's Rules of Engagement

1. Prepare thoroughly for your mission.
   If your mission fails, it will most likely result from lack of understanding of the country, the culture, or from inadequate team preparation and leadership.
2. Learn the local culture.
   Absence of cultural knowledge at minimum is equivalent to disrespect. At worst, it may be harmful to your patients and lethal to your program.
3. Learn survival language.
   Knowing the local language will make you less isolated, more effective, and may even help you survive.
4. Learn triage skills—for both patients and problems.
   A well-trained triage officer not only can manage a large number of direct cases but also will seek to identify indirect cases that may signal an emerging public health crisis.

D. A. Bradt, C. M. Drummond, *Pocket Field Guide for Disaster Health Professionals*,
https://doi.org/10.1007/978-3-030-04801-3

5. Learn mental health skills.
   They will help you better understand your patients as well as yourself. Be an active listener. Listen more than you talk. Remember the most common presenting complaint will be a mental health one. A patient's mental health status reveals what trauma came beforehand.
6. Improve your physical diagnosis skills.
   Western trained clinicians rely on labs and x-rays which won't be available. Clinical decisions will be made on the accuracy of your physical exam and the "decoding" of vital signs.
7. Gather data on outcomes.
   We need to know and document health outcomes—what we did, why we did it, to whom we did it, and whether it did any good—in order to educate the next generation of humanitarians. Write up your experiences for others as well as yourself.
8. Schedule adequate time for sleep and leave. Beware of fatigue, drugs, and alcohol.
   Providers of acute trauma care should be high on your list for concern.
9. Establish personal friendships.
   Let these friendships be outlets for your personal and professional frustrations. While it's important to keep your own counsel, the more you can verbalize your frustration, the less harm you bring to your patients.
10. Master the 3 most adaptive defense mechanisms: resilience, acceptance, sense of humor.
    Stress management skills and coping strategies can improve the odds of a healthy outcome from disaster.
11. Provide leadership.
    Difficult or impossible leadership decisions will be the norm. Make them. But don't play God. Ask your team members for their input. Good, fair and shared leadership will result in better health outcomes.
12. Know how and when to delegate.
    Leaders may or may not make friends within their chain of command, but they must be able to delegate.
13. Practice humility.
    It's a good antidote to power intoxication.
14. Dare to be creative.
    It will be some of your best work. But don't promise or do anything that cannot be duplicated by the host country healthcare providers after you leave.

Adapted by the authors from personal communication with Skip Burkle, Oct 11, 2016, and from Burkle FM. Coping with stress under conditions of disaster and refugee care. *Mil Med* 1983; 148:800–3. Used with permission.

Judy Lee's Rules of Engagement

1. Have a solid base of support at home.
   Reduce or eliminate worry over bill payments, schedule conflicts, and spousal separation, etc.
2. Travel to an assignment with as much information as possible.
   Ask questions about the type and scope of the disaster. Know what to expect and plan for it before you arrive on site. Mission essentials are: proper mission definition along with details of the disaster, assignment of key leadership personnel, and full commitment of resources required to fulfill the mission.
3. Travel light.
   Be prepared to carry your own luggage. Peanut butter and crackers may be all you get for awhile.
4. Know the team members.
   Get to know any colleagues you don't already know en route or as soon as possible on arrival. Relying on each other will be key.
5. Be flexible—willing to work in an area of need that is not your original assignment.
   Florence Nightingale went to Crimea to care for war casualties and was assigned to medical supply.
6. Respect the work of others on the team not in the health field.
   There are necessary functions others fulfill in disaster management: accounting, human resources, logistics, etc. They are there to help you carry out your work.
7. See the big picture.
   See the whole picture to the extent possible—the whole patient, the whole family, the whole disaster. Women who do so will surpass those male colleagues who think only of finances, regulations, and machismo rather than humanity.
8. Keep notes on key issues and daily actions.
   A regular daily log will make reporting easier and preserve a record of actions you might otherwise not readily recall.
9. Teach as you go.
   Pass on disaster preparedness keys so that if there is a next time, mitigation can take place. You won't always be there, so help the locals to integrate and work with future incoming staff. Remember, they remain even after you leave.
10. Stay balanced in the field.
    Pace yourself, keep a sense of humor, make new connections, renew old friendships, get your rest, and detach periodically.
11. Know your limitations.

Don't overextend yourself and risk becoming a part of the disaster rather than the solution. Be prepared to evacuate (others) and demission (yourself) as circumstances require.

12. Accept the need to continually train and prepare.
    Preparation is the best way to stay functional and indeed thrive in the stress of the field. Conferences, classes, standards, and regulations, including those of partner agencies, are within your scope of responsibility. You have to like the details.
13. Be able to sell your superiors on important policy issues when they cannot see the added value.
    Disaster mental health and disaster logistics were among the core concepts initially resisted by bureaucrats of the day. Involve the right people, compile the latest literature, accumulate data, and engage with your colleagues.
14. Read about inspiring and effective predecessors.
    Clara Barton, Jane Delano, and Florence Nightingale all changed the disaster world. You can too.

Adapted by the authors from personal communication with Judy Lee, Mar 3, 2017. Used with permission.

Tom Durant's Rules of Engagement

1. The purpose of the mission is humanitarian health assistance.
   Not data gathering for academic researchers, report writing for agency donors, or media relations for advocacy groups.
2. The work of the medical coordinator is beneficiary care.
   Corporate communications, accounting, and administration are all important, but if you are not directly serving refugees, then you are not touching those most in need.
3. Understand each other.
   Listen to people fully. Speak to people respectfully. People are sometimes the problem and always the solution. If you don't understand the people, then you don't understand either the problem or the solution.
4. Understand the complexity of refugee medicine.
   The best clinicians in refugee medicine know what supersedes their clinical work—most importantly, security and public health. You must understand those sectors in order to best run your clinical operation.
5. Don't re-invent the wheel.
   Read the work of your predecessors.
6. Don't make promises.
   When in doubt—observe, measure, and think (OMT). You can always be a good listener.
7. Don't sweat the small stuff.

Wisdom comes from experience. Experience comes from mistakes. You will make them.

8. The biggest pitfall is arrogance.
   The best docs are able to say "I don't know", "I made a mistake", "I'm sorry", and "Thank you". Tom was hardest on himself. At M&M of cases from "unidentified" practitioners, Tom would publicly criticize his own clinical judgment.
9. The biggest asset is humor—even more than intelligence.
   Make friends and disarm enemies with humor. A joke on you is the best. Otherwise, Irish and rugby stories are preferred.
10. There are a lot of heroes out there. Find one and work with her.
    Most of the heroes are the refugees themselves, and most of those are women. They will generally be anonymous. Some of the ex-pat heroes in Goma were San Francisco fire fighters who provided clean water from pumper trucks, and Goal volunteers who buried the dead.
11. Stay the course.
    If you haven't been in the field for at least several months, then you are a medical tourist. If you stay long enough, you will experience predictable phases in your project. The classic ones are: enthusiasm, disillusionment, panic, search for the guilty, punishment of the innocent, then praise and honor for the non-participants.
12. Stay out of politics.
    Pinstripe is the most dangerous camouflage in the jungle. You need to understand politics but not to change it. Your job is to help your organization and its program beneficiaries—not to change the organization much less the health system in which it operates.
13. Do not be afraid.
    Any fear you face is likely a fraction of the fear refugees have lived with. Don't make a big deal about it. Get on with the job. If you are in a combat situation, then you may have to be a little brave. You do it five minutes at a time. Ultimately, you must anticipate, adapt, or die.

Adapted by the authors from personal communication with Tom Durant deceased Oct 30, 2001.

About the Authors

David A. Bradt, MD, MPH, FACEP, FACEM, FAFPHM, DTM&H is a specialist in emergency medicine and public health. He trained at academic medical centers in the USA, the UK, and Australia as well as cross-trained in disaster management through the ICRC, WHO, the UNHCR, and the USAID/OFDA. His field experience includes disaster response in 25 countries and territories. He served as emergency physician in the Mujahideen-Afghan Surgical Hospital at the Afghan-Pakistan border during the Afghan-Soviet war, International Federation of Red Cross and Red Crescent Societies medical coordinator in Zaire during the Rwandan genocide, International Rescue Committee physician in Macedonia and Albania during the Kosovo ethnic cleansing, WHO medical coordinator in Indonesia after the Indian Ocean tsunami, WHO emergency coordinator in Tunisia during the Libyan civil war, WHO senior public health advisor in South Sudan during its civil war, USAID/OFDA senior field officer in Sudan during the Darfur genocide, USAID/OFDA health advisor to the US Interagency Task Force after the Haiti earthquake, USAID/OFDA regional advisor in Southern Africa during the El Niño drought, and American Red Cross medical consultant at US disasters including World Trade Center terrorism.

Dr. Bradt is a Rockefeller Foundation Bellagio Center resident scholar, a John Simon Guggenheim Memorial Foundation fellow, and a Fulbright specialist in public/global health. He has received multiple awards for disaster response including the International Federation for Emergency Medicine Humanitarian Award.

Christina M. Drummond, AM, MBBS, FRACP, FAFPHM, MPH, MAE, DObst (RCOG), DTM&H is a specialist in infectious diseases and public health. She trained at academic medical centers in Australia, the USA, and the UK as well as cross-trained in disaster management and disease control

D. A. Bradt, C. M. Drummond, *Pocket Field Guide for Disaster Health Professionals*,
https://doi.org/10.1007/978-3-030-04801-3

through the ICRC, WHO, and the US CDC. Her field experience includes service in 24 countries and territories. She served as Australian Red Cross medical team leader in Cambodia during the Khmer Rouge insurgency, International Federation of Red Cross medical coordinator in Zaire during the Rwandan genocide, American Red Cross epidemiologist in Guam after Supertyphoon Paka, International Rescue Committee physician in Macedonia and Albania during the Kosovo ethnic cleansing, WHO medical officer for tuberculosis in Indonesia during the Timor crisis, UNICEF-CDC technical advisor for Stop Polio in Sudan, CARE International health project manager in Sudan during the Darfur genocide, WHO consultant in the Maldives and in India after the Indian Ocean tsunami, WHO public health consultant in Cambodia after Mekong River flooding, and Medecins Sans Frontieres-Holland infectious diseases advisor.

Dr. Drummond is a Rockefeller Foundation Bellagio Center resident scholar. She has received multiple awards for her humanitarian work including an Order of Australia.

About the Society

The Disaster Medical Coordination International Society is a private, nonprofit, operational, technical, humanitarian organization based in Washington, DC, which works to save lives through evidence-based best practices in disaster management and humanitarian assistance.
The Society endorses the following principled vision of health professionals in disasters:

- Professionalization of health personnel in disasters requires apprenticeship training, code of ethics, continuing education, and peer review.
- Qualifications for health professionals are competency-based, criterion-referenced, and time-limited.
- Competency is case-related—extensive field experience is fundamental to disaster expertise.
- Expertise in the disaster health sector is specialty-specific, site-specific, hazard-specific, and organization-specific.

State of the art in the disaster health sector emerges from interdisciplinary, interagency, and international best practices.

D. A. Bradt, C. M. Drummond, *Pocket Field Guide for Disaster Health Professionals*,
https://doi.org/10.1007/978-3-030-04801-3

Index

D. A. Bradt, C. M. Drummond, *Pocket Field Guide for Disaster Health Professionals*,
https://doi.org/10.1007/978-3-030-04801-3

The manufacturer's authorised representative in the EU is Springer Nature Customer Service Centre GmbH, Europaplatz 3, 69115 Heidelberg, Germany. If you have any concerns regarding our products, please contact ProductSafety@springernature.com

Printed and bound by CPI Group (UK) Ltd, Croydon, CR0 4YY
01/10/2026
02226299-0001

The manufacturer's authorised representative in the EU is Springer Nature Customer Service Centre GmbH, Europaplatz 3, 69115 Heidelberg, Germany. If you have any concerns regarding our products, please contact ProductSafety@springernature.com

Printed and bound by CPI Group (UK) Ltd, Croydon, CR0 4YY
01/10/2026
02226299-0001